How to Enjoy a Healthy Family

HOW · TO · FAMILY
SERIES

How to

Enjoy

a

Healthy

Family

Even in Stressful Times

Bobbie Reed, Ph.D.

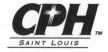

How to Family Series

How to Be a Great First-Time Father
How to Be Together on Sunday Morning
How to Enjoy a Healthy Family
    (Even in Stressful Times)

Unless otherwise noted, Scripture quotations are taken from THE HOLY BIBLE, NEW INTERNATION VERSION®. Copyright © 1973, 1978, 1984 by the International Bible Society. Used by permission of Zondervan Publishing House. All rights reserved.

The "NIV" and "New International Version" trademarks are registered in the United States Patent and Trademark Office by the International Bible Society. Use of either trademark requires the permission of the International Bible Society.

Copyright © 1995 Concordia Publishing House
3558 S. Jefferson Avenue, St. Louis, MO 63118-3968
Manufactured in the United States of America

Library of Congress Cataloging-in-Publication Data.

Reed, Bobbie.
    How to enjoy a healthy family: even in stressful times / Bobbie Reed.
        p.   cm.   — (How to family series)
    Includes bibliographical references.
    ISBN 0-570-04691-2
    1. Family—Religious life. 2. Family—United States. 3. Christian life.
    4. Family—Health and hygiene. 5. Stress (Psychology)—Religious
aspects—Christianity. I. Title. II. Series.
BV456.2.R42 1995
248.4—dc20   94-39362

1 2 3 4 5 6 7 8 9 10   04 03 02 01 00 99 98 97 96 95

To Pamela Bines,
with love and appreciation,
for being a significant person in
my supportive network,
and someone who helps me cope
when times get stressful.

CONTENTS

❦ As You Begin: Life Is Stressful

"If one more thing goes wrong, I'm going to go stark, raving mad!"

"I'm at the end of my rope!"

"I just can't take any more!"

Do these statements sound familiar? Most of us have made similar comments at various times in our lives, signaling that we are experiencing stress overload. Learning how to effectively cope with extreme or constant stress has become an almost absolute requirement in today's hurry-scurry world. Understanding the nature of stress is an important prerequisite to building effective coping strengths in your life.

People comment that their colleague has been under a lot of stress when a co-worker is hospitalized after a heart attack. Tension headaches are attributed to stress. Executives admit to being under stress when faced with too many demands and too few resources.

While these concepts are not totally erroneous, they are based on the premise that stress is an external force over which the individual has little control. A look at the clinical definition of stress, and an investigation of the research findings, reveals the surprising truth that stress is actually a combination of two factors: a stressor and the response—sometimes called stress reactivity. If there is no stress reactivity, there is no stress. This is why it is possible for two individuals to experience the same situation and one becomes stressed while the other does not. Note: When a stressor causes you an uncomfortable response, you are experiencing stress.

There are three basic categories of stressors that we will explore in detail in chapter 1: *change, challenge,* and *conflict.* You may have problems coping with only one of these types of stressors, or you may find two or three difficult. Whichever the case, it will be wise to take a look at how you respond to changes, challenges, and conflicts, because these three stressors are inevitable in life.

The good news is that the Jesus who loved you enough to die for you has felt every bit of stress we experience. With His help and presence, you will learn to control the discomfort. This book will present information to assist you in reducing, and even preventing, your stress reactivity. The first step is learning about the physiology of stress reactivity and identifying the symptoms you experience when under stress. Next will come a conscious effort to eliminate as many stressors in your life as you can. Learning how to control your own response to stressors is also a critical step. But, perhaps, the most significant action you will take is developing coping strengths. The more stress you have, the stronger you will need to be physically, spiritually, mentally, psychologically, and socially. Your stress can help you discover and develop your strength.

Jesus understood that life can be stressful. He gave us good guidelines to follow.

- When you are weary and feeling burdened, He invites you to come to Him. He will give you rest (Matt. 11:28).

- He says, do not let your heart be troubled, but trust in Him and His ability to care for you (John 14:1).

- When you get worried about making ends meet—feeding and clothing yourself (and by extension, your family)—you can remember that God is in control and cares for you. Ask His Spirit to help you put the Almighty first in your life, and trust Him for the rest (Matt. 6:25–33).

- Paul continues God's message. He admonishes you to not be anxious for anything, but to bring your requests to God in prayer (Phil. 4:6–7).

- Peter reminds you to cast all of your cares and

worries upon the Lord, because He cares for you (1 Peter 5:7).

The message is clear: You do not have to live a life controlled by stress. In spite of the fact that life is stressful, you don't have to be stressed out! This book can help. God will help.

PART I: UNDERSTAND STRESS AND DISTRESS

1 RECOGNIZE STRESS

I was waiting for my interview for a job promotion, but I had very ambivalent feelings. I knew I was qualified, had prepared well, and was ready for the increased responsibility. I liked the idea of being pushed (challenged) beyond my comfort zone and being given an opportunity to prove what I could do. On the other hand, the new position would require me to live away from my family during the week for the next several months. The idea of finding a different place to live and learning where everything was in the new community felt intimidating. The changes would be significant. Finally, the new position involved following a predecessor whose management and operational style were in direct conflict with my own.

Considering that this promotion would provide the three major types of stressors—change, challenge, and conflict—in abundance, you can readily understand that I was torn between wanting the promotion and hoping I didn't get it. (I got it.)

What Are Stressors?

If you are serious about wanting to begin to reduce the stress in your life and control your stress reactivity, the first step will be to identify the stressors you face. Let's look at the three types of stressors.

- Change.

    Any change is a potential stressor, yet change is a fact of life. Political liaisons are formed and broken in quick succession. New technology and research affect our lives daily. New or improved products appear on the supermarket shelves. Other products are taken off shelves because they have been found to be potentially dangerous to our health. We learn a new version of a computer program only to discover that, just when we are comfortable with it, it has been upgraded. Each year thousands of laws are passed, regulations adopted, and court decisions made that impact our daily lives and our businesses.

    Our *social* world changes. Close friends move away. A co-worker is promoted. A neighbor dies. The "ideal" marriage ends in divorce. Our children enter junior high school where, in some communities, sex and drugs become readily available.

Some changes are *career* related. We transfer, are promoted, or change jobs. New discoveries in our professional disciplines quickly make skills we've learned obsolete. We must keep learning.

Each day, as you cope with these demands, you initiate your own changes. You grow and develop new knowledge, new skills, or new abilities. You begin a diet, upgrade your lifestyle, or assume new financial obligations.

Each change in our lives triggers a physiological response, however slight. You are constantly processing responses to the thousands of stressors you experience each day. Much of the time you are unaware of either the stressor (as such) or of your responses because the body functions so automatically. However, if an accumulation of small stressors keeps adding up, if a stressor persists for too long or increases in intensity, your stress reactivity can rise to an uncomfortable level.

Consider, for example, entering a dimly lit room and turning on a lamp. You may not be aware of the adjustment your pupils make to the additional light. However, if you were in a very dark room and someone repeatedly turned a bright light off and on, your body's response would be increased, and you would probably begin to feel discomfort. You might become agitated.

A major change in your life can prove very stressful, even if everything else has been going along very well. A spouse announcing, "I want a divorce"; a death in the family; sudden bankruptcy; a major loss; a serious accident, injury or illness; or some other life shock can immediately send a person into seemingly unbearable stress reactivity and overload.

- Challenge.

Also in the stressor category are demands that push you beyond your physical, emotional, or psychological comfort zone. It is exciting to stretch a little beyond your reach, but it's stressful if the stretch is too far.

It is fun to try a new skill, attempt to negotiate a better deal with a tough salesperson, or accomplish a seemingly impossible task at work within an unreasonable deadline. But if there is an expectation that unreasonable demands and deadlines will continue over a long period of time, the stress becomes much more difficult to handle. Almost anyone can work a 12-hour day once every six months to get a special project done. But working 12 hours a day, every day, seven days a week will eventually become too stressful, physically.

Most of us will respond with sympathy and comfort if one of our friends comes crying to us with a major life problem. But if several of our friends are asking for care, and if our children are also demanding our attention, and if our spouse gets sick and requires special patience, our emotional strength will eventually run out. Being needed becomes another stressor.

If you are not meeting your own personal expectations for yourself, or if you are aware that you are not meeting the expectations of others, you can also feel additional stress.

• Conflict.

Whenever one person's choices or inner thrust runs counter to another person's values, needs, wants, plans, or inner thrust, conflict results. And since none of us is a carbon copy of another, conflict is inevitable. Conflict, in itself, is neither good nor bad. It does, however, present an opportunity to interact with another human being to bring about resolution. How that interaction is handled is the significant aspect that often causes conflict. For most people, conflict is a stressor. Some people can confront another individual productively without a second thought because they have learned appropriate skills. But unless you have learned these skills, chances are you will have difficulty with conflict situations.

Also in the category of conflict are any real or perceived threats to our physical, emotional, or psychological safety. All threats are stressors. If you are walking down a dark street and hear footsteps approaching you from behind, you may become fearful and experience stress. If someone rejects you or says something you find hurtful, you may become stressed. If you believe that a co-worker is going to get a promotion that you believe should be yours, or if you are belittled or criticized, you may experience a stress response. The response can occur whether the threat is actual or merely anticipated.

Stressors tend to accumulate to create major stress reactivity. One or two small stressors will not usually cause a major stress reaction, unless they continue over a long period of time. A small change (such as turning a light on and off), if continued over a period of time, can cause significant stress reactivity. Several small changes, none of which would be major stressors by themselves, occurring within a short period of time can cause uncomfortable stress reactivity. For example: You get up late; you discover you don't have food in the house to pack for lunch; you get stuck in traffic; the boss asks you about an overdue report; a co-worker spills coffee on your paperwork; you get a telephone call from the principal of your daughter's school asking for an appointment—soon; and you remember that you forgot to leave a roast out to thaw for dinner. If all of these things happened within a couple of hours, you would probably experience significant stress reactivity.

Of course, you would not want to live without any stressors. Life without change would be boring and uneventful. You would not grow and learn. You would not form interactive relationships. You would not stretch to meet new goals and achieve new heights in your career or personal or spiritual life. Your response to stressors can provide a positive force in your life if you choose to be challenged by them and if you learn to deal with them appropriately.

What Is the Stress Response?

Our bodies are made to produce bursts of power and energy as a response to stressors we encounter. This is called a stress response or stress reactivity. Your body will become physiologically prepared to either stay and fight or run away. This is called the "fight-flight syndrome." If the stressor is purely physical, one of these two choices might be appropriate and the stress reactivity useful. As you either run or fight, your body uses up the extra physical energy generated by the fight-flight syndrome and gradually returns to normal functioning.

However, in today's society, most of the stressors are emotional, psychological, or mental, and therefore, fighting or fleeing are not usually the appropriate choices. Consequently, the extra energy generated by the fight-flight syndrome is not used up and causes physiological problems. Let's take a closer look at this.

Fight-Flight Syndrome

Hans Selye (*The Stress of Life*, Rev. ed. New York: McGraw-Hill, Inc., 1976) explains that there are three stages to the fight-flight syndrome, which we will call stress reactivity. The first stage is *alarm*. In this stage, your heart pounds rapidly—pumping additional blood through the body and increasing blood pressure. Breathing becomes more rapid to increase the flow of oxygen into the systems. Your metabolic rate rises to more easily convert stored energy into usable energy, and additional hormones are secreted into your system to assist in this conversion of energy. Your body's blood supply is diverted away from the fine motor muscles to the large muscles (reducing coordination, temperature, and feeling in the extremities). Sight and hearing become more sensitive. "Unnecessary" systems, such as the digestive and immune systems, are temporarily shut down. Your skeletal muscles brace for action, and because the brain is concentrating on physical action, abstract reasoning becomes difficult.

In this first stage, the body is highly charged with energy—the muscles are braced for immediate action. Your awareness is heightened to detect any additional dangers that may be lurking undiscovered. You are ready for major action.

David, the psalmist, says in Psalm 139:14, we are fearfully and wonderfully made. If you are faced with physical dangers and need to fight off wild animals, enemies, or even a falling tree limb, you need additional physical strength. God designed your body to automatically produce the energy needed to face these dangers. Therefore, these body changes are valuable when you need to exert an increased degree of physical energy. The amazing thing is that these bodily changes can occur as quickly as eight seconds after the triggering event, and even more quickly if the stressor is significant enough. Think of the last time a car cut in front of you unexpectedly. Remember how you felt that shot of adrenaline accompanied by the instant slamming on the brakes? It probably didn't take eight seconds to act.

The second stage is called *resistance*. When the stressor continues over a period of time, the body adapts to the need for producing increased energy and uses the energy to meet the additional physical demands. Under the pressure of a deadline (stressor), students can study long hours and get by on less sleep for a few days. Their bodies, through the stress reactivity process, produce the additional energy needed. The length of time persons can remain in the resistance stage is determined by a variety of factors—physical conditioning, emotional stability, psychological wholeness, spiritual strength, and coping abilities. Eventually, if the stressor is not removed or the stress reactivity is not reduced, the person will move to stage 3.

Stage 3 is called *exhaustion*. When there is prolonged exposure to stressors, the body's ability to maintain itself at the resistance stage will become depleted. A person in this stage becomes physically, emotionally, psychologically, and spiritually exhausted. If there is no relief, the person will become ill and can even die.

The very coping mechanism God gave us to deal with unexpected dangers can become a threat if you ignore the warning signals and fail to take appropriate action.

Your Stress

What is the level of stress in your life? Before you read further, you might want to work through the Social Readjustment Rating Scale quiz (Appendix A). This will help you assess the changes that may have had an impact on your life within the last 12 months.

After taking the quiz, make a list of the following:.

1. Any anticipated changes or perceived threats to your physical, emotional, psychological, or spiritual well-being.

2. Any unresolved hurts, rejections, or relationships.

3. Any area in your life where you are being challenged or pushed beyond your limits (physically, emotionally, psychologically, or spiritually).

4. Any conflicts that you have failed to resolve or will face during the next two weeks.

Taking the quiz and listing anticipated stressors will give you an idea of the level of stress you are experiencing. If you want an even better profile, record your feelings during the next three weeks. Note each time you feel upset, fearful, stressed, challenged, or confronted. Record times when you experience stress reactivity. List each event and your response—physical, emotional, and intellectual. (What did you do? How did you feel? What did you say or tell yourself about that event?)

Don't be discouraged if you discover a high number of stressors in your life. There is hope. With the help of God's Holy Spirit, *you can* increase your ability to cope. The secret to coping with stress in the family is to understand stress and stress reactivity. Recognize the stressors you face. Learn to reduce your stress reactivity or to use up the excess energy as it is produced and no longer needed. You must learn how to function as a transformer—divert the extra energy, step down the available energy, and maintain only the amount of energy needed to enjoy your daily life. The Spirit can help you *transform your stress into strength.*

2
Develop Coping Strengths

Remember the last time you attempted to sit or stand on something that would not support your weight—an old chair, a wooden box, or a small table? As you placed your weight on the object, creaking and cracking sounds probably warned you that there was an imminent danger of collapse. If you immediately raised off the object, there was probably no harm done. However, if you ignored the warnings, chances are the item broke and you ended up falling to the floor, perhaps injuring yourself in the process. This is a fairly accurate analogy of a human being experiencing stress that exceeds the coping strength.

When your stress exceeds your strength, you initially go into an "overdrive" condition. Your body, through the stress reactivity response, produces the extra energy you need to cope beyond your normal strength. (This is the "resistance" stage discussed in chapter 1.) This "resistance" allows you to function for a short period of time, during which you receive warning signals—signs that you are nearing a breaking point. If you ignore these signals, you will likely proceed to the "exhaustion" stage—and experience a complete inability to cope.

To carry the analogy through, imagine what would happen if you simply plopped down on an unsteady table, box, or chair. The creaking, cracking, and collapse would occur simultaneously. A sudden and severe stressor that exceeds a person's ability to cope can cause immediate inability to function.

Some people seem able to endure incredibly stressful situations and continue to function productively, while others collapse at the slightest problem. What makes the difference? The same thing that makes the difference in the ability of small items to bear heavy weights—the strength of the item. A small stool made of balsa wood will collapse even under a small child's weight, while a small stool made of oak can support a fully grown adult. The material from which an item is made, or the manner in which it is reinforced, will determine its ability to handle different challenges. Human beings are no different.

There are five areas of life in which God can help you develop coping strengths. Developing strength in these areas will help you to cope better with everyday stressors as well as the unexpected and undesirable challenges life may bring. These areas include the physical, spiritual, mental, psychological, and social. Failure to develop adequate coping strengths in these areas will leave you open to the five deadly "Ds": disease, defeat, distress, depression, and desertion.

Develop Physical Strength to Avoid Disease

God designed your body to respond to your environment and adjust appropriately. If the outside temperature is too hot, your body gears up an extra cooling system and you begin to perspire. If your body has an infection, white blood cells increase to fight off the attack. If light is too bright, the pupils of your eyes constrict. Under stress reactivity, your body temporarily abandons many of the autonomic systems in order to produce the extra energy you need to cope. As long as this stage is brief, no permanent or serious harm is done to the body. However, if there is prolonged exposure to continued stress, and the body continues in the resistance mode, physical problems can develop.

- Because stress reactivity pulls blood away from the stomach and slows or shuts down the digestive system, a prolonged resistance stage can result in digestive problems—ulcers, colitis, spastic colons, constipation, or diarrhea.

- Because stress reactivity causes the muscles to brace, a prolonged resistance stage can result in back and shoulder spasms, tension headaches, and temporo-mandibular (TMJ) syndrome (jaw clenching).

- Because stress reactivity causes blood to be drawn away from the extremities, there can be increased injuries because of a lack of coordination of fine motor muscles (e.g. fingers). There may also be increased dermatological problems and constant cold/clammy hands and feet.

- Because stress reactivity is believed to temporarily slow down the body's immune system, a prolonged resistance stage leaves a person more susceptible to germs and viruses.

- The additional stress placed on the heart and the increased blood pressure involved in a prolonged stress reactivity can cause heart attacks, perpetual high blood pressure, or strokes.

It is easily seen that while the stress response is a positive gift from God, He intended it for a specific and short-term function—not as a way of life. The body cannot healthily exist in a constant state of stress reactivity.

If you have not taken care of your physical condition, your body may not be able to cope with even a small amount of stress. Even if you are reasonably healthy, there are ways you can increase your physical coping strength so that you can endure the usual stressors of life as well as the unexpected shocks.

Steps to becoming physically strong

• Eat a balanced diet, high in fiber, low in fat.

Make eating properly a way of life. Instead of fad diets, study nutrition and carefully select the foods you eat. Fresh fruits and vegetables (at least three servings a day) are desirable. Select chicken, turkey, or fish over red meat whenever possible.

Limit your intake of refined sugars and starches (white bread, for example). It is believed that digesting refined sugars and starches, as well as alcohol, depletes the body of the vitamins it needs to process the glucose generated by stress reactivity.

Avoid stimulants such as caffeine and nicotine, because they force the body into a pseudo-stress reactivity response by increasing the production of glucose.

Daniel, of Old Testament fame, had a personal eating plan that he refused to change—even when asked to eat at the king's table. God blessed Daniel (and his friends) for sticking to their proper eating plan (Dan. 1:5–15). Ask God to help you and your family develop healthy food habits as well. It is easier to stick with an eating plan than to "live on a diet."

- Maintain a proper weight level.

    You may not be able to achieve your desired weight as indicated by your doctors' charts, but set a goal to work toward that weight. Imagine strapping a 25-pound bag of flour to your back and carrying it around all day. In much the same way, excess pounds can drain your physical coping strength. The more overweight you are, the less able to handle additional stress.

- Drink lots of water.

    A simple thing—drinking lots of water each day—can make a great difference in your physical well-being. Nutritionists recommend a minimum of eight glasses of water a day (64 oz.). Drinking water increases efficient functioning of the body.

- Exercise.

    Think of exercising as a way to tune up your body and develop its coping strength. Proper exercise increases the body's metabolism rate, develops muscles and keeps them toned, keeps the body flexible, and uses up some of the stress reactivity energy produced when the body is under stress.

- Get enough sleep.

You can function for a while on less sleep than you truly need, but eventually your body will no longer be alert and at its best. Determine the number of hours per night you need in order to function productively. Start by setting a specific bedtime—say 10 o'clock. Set your alarm for six o'clock. This will allow you eight hours of sleep. Follow this routine for a week. Then either go to bed one half hour later or set your alarm one half hour earlier (depending upon whether you are a "night" or a "morning" person). Follow that schedule for a week. Keep shortening your sleeping time by one half hour a week until your body tells you that you have eliminated too much sleep. Return to the prior week's schedule. Plan your schedule so that you get your full night's sleep.

Another goal is to make your sleep as restful as possible. If your mind is reluctant to let go of problems and you find you dream about them all night, try reading an engrossing or entertaining book before you go to sleep. This will interrupt your worry. Or use the time before you go to bed to meditate on a particularly restful or comforting Scripture passage. Spend time in prayer, turning your problems over to God. It may also help to take a warm bath, do relaxation exercises, or go for a long walk.

- Relax.

    When the body is under stress, the muscles brace, ready to run or fight. It is often necessary to consciously relax. At the office you can stop work for a few minutes and force each muscle group to unbrace and relax. Roll your head from side to side. Hunch your shoulders and let them totally relax. "Shake out" your arms and legs. If these exercises are done three or four times a day, you can avoid muscles spasms that result from prolonged body tension.

    At home, lie on the floor and totally tense up your entire body, including the muscles in your face. Hold the tension for about five seconds, then totally relax every part of the body. Do this several times to learn the difference between tension and relaxation. After you are familiar with the difference, you can begin to consciously relax each set of muscles in the body—one group at a time. Tensing and relaxing for 10 to 20 minutes is a great way to rid the body of unnecessary muscular tension.

- Do something enjoyable.

    One thing you can do to help your body retain its resiliency is to vary your activity. You will want to plan your leisure activities to counterbalance your working activities. If you have a desk job, then perhaps a physically active leisure choice would be wise. If your job is physically demanding, you may enjoy sedentary activities such as playing table games, playing the piano, or attending sports events or the symphony. If your job involves a lot of people contact, your leisure preference might include reading, writing, or other quiet, solitary activities. If you seldom have contact with others at work, your leisure choices will probably include more social interaction.

Whether or not you vary your activity, it is important to include in your schedule some time to do things you personally enjoy and find rewarding. If you are a single parent, working and taking care of the home and children, your available free time may be limited. Use your time wisely and make time for yourself.

In the Bible, God tells us to take care of our bodies. In Old Testament times, God gave specific dietary laws to protect the Israelites from serious illnesses. In the New Testament, God reminds us that our bodies are the temples of the Holy Spirit and belong to God. God invites us to present our bodies as living sacrifices to Him. God enables us to give Him glory whether we eat or drink or whatever we do (Rom. 12:1; 1 Cor. 6:19–20; 1 Cor. 10:31). Taking care of the physical body is an important spiritual activity and responsibility.

Warning signals

Each of these seven suggestions can help you develop increased physical coping strength. Even so, it is important that you become aware of and respond to warnings that signal the end of your physical strength. These signals remind you to reduce the stressors in your life and increase your activity in the area of physical conditioning. If you don't resolve the problem (stressor and/or poor physical conditioning), you may eventually find that your body has given way to a serious disease.

Do you have frequent headaches, backaches, colds, allergies, flu symptoms, infections, heartburn, stomach pain, diarrhea, constipation, insomnia, fatigue, restlessness, or minor aches and pains in various parts of the body? These quite possibly are the warning signals your body is sending to let you know that action is needed. Do not ignore them. Do not become diseased.

Depend on God's Strength to Avoid Defeat

In Ephesians 6:10–13, Paul tells us to carefully gird ourselves with spiritual armor in order to withstand life's daily pressures. We need God's armor to fend off spiritual attacks from Satan and his followers. We have within ourselves a propensity to sin. Sin separates us from God and saps our spiritual strength.

God's Holy Spirit works faith in us. We depend on His power and motivation to help us trust and obey God. Ask the Holy Spirit to increase your spiritual strength as you prayerfully consider the following steps.

Steps to spiritual coping strength

- Do right.

  In Paul's analogy of the Christian soldier (Eph. 6:12–17), the breastplate represents obedience—doing right. When you let Jesus help you make the right choices, when through His power you follow God's commands, your heart is protected from the enemy's attacks. Jesus said that by abiding in Him, you are able to keep His commandments and show that you love Him. Jesus' love and power gives you the strength to walk close by His side each day (cf. John 15:10).

- Be truthful.

  Honesty is the best policy, even when it's not the easiest choice. Ask God to help you be honest in all your dealings—to make your word as good as your bond. Then people will quickly learn they can trust you. God can strengthen your personal integrity and help you be true to what you believe. He can help you keep promises, even to yourself. When you are honest before God, you are more able to see yourself as you are seen, and if you don't like what you see, God can help you change (Rom. 12:2–3). Truth is a critical piece of the Christian's armor (Eph. 6:14).

- Be at peace.

What a strange admonition for a person living in a stressful world! Yet Jesus was able to lie down in a boat and sleep while a storm raged (Mark 4:35–41). The disciples were not at peace. They were afraid—first because of the storm's power, later because of the power Jesus displayed in quieting the storm.

Most of us are like the disciples—fearful, regardless of which way the wind blows. Take another look at the disciples in the boat. Can't you hear the terrified anger in their voices as they waken Jesus: "We are all going to die! Don't you care?" Sometimes our fears are expressed in anger too. We are afraid we aren't getting the respect, recognition, or assistance we deserve, and we become angry. We not only become involved in needless conflict, we often generate it ourselves! Paul reminds us that God's armor offers peace (Eph. 6:15).

- Pray regularly.

God is our salvation. He saved us from eternal condemnation and promises to guard us against Satan's daily attacks. Be in constant contact with your Lord through prayer. Paul encourages us to pray without ceasing (1 Thess. 5:17).

When you are in tune with God, you can have the attitude of Christ (Phil. 2:5). As you pray, the Holy Spirit will help you remember things you have read in the Word of God. He will help you make right choices, trust God, and respond appropriately to sinful situations (John 14:26). When you start your day with prayer, and continue to touch base with God throughout the hours, you will find that problems are easier to deal with because you have a conquering partner assisting you. Greater is the One in you than the one in the world (Rom. 8:31–39; 1 John 4:4).

Paul calls the mental armor or protection the helmet of salvation (Eph. 6:17). God is our salvation. Keep in touch with your protector.

- Know your Bible.

The Word of God, the Bible, is the Christian's sword (Eph. 6:17). Jesus used Scripture to rebuke Satan when tempted in the wilderness

(Matt. 4:1–11). Each time Satan tried a new temptation, Jesus began His answer with the words "it is written ...," and finally Satan left Jesus. He could not stand against the Scripture's power. Jesus helps us search the Scriptures to find the way to eternal life and peace. The Spirit works through the Bible to lead us to Christ (John 5:39).

Just reading the Bible is not enough. Ask God to help you study His Word. Reflect on it. Absorb it. Internalize and act upon it. The better you know Scriptures, the more you meditate on and search God's Word, the more opportunities the Spirit has to strengthen you spiritually. Memorizing significant verses will be a big help in this process. Then ask God to help you be "a doer of the Word" (James 1:22–25).

• Be built up in Christ.

The Holy Spirit will strengthen you as you follow these five steps, but two additional things can also help.

First, fellowship with other believers. Fellowship means more than just belonging to a group, attending a meeting with other believers, or going to church. Fellowship means getting together to interact and encourage one another (Heb. 10:25). When you lag behind, or feel weak, let a brother or sister in Christ encourage you. When you are feeling strong, encourage someone else. There is strength in numbers. It is easy to snap in half a single twig. But if you tightly bind a hundred twigs together, it becomes very difficult, or even impossible, to break one.

Second, collect "faith memorials." In the Old Testament, God told the Israelites to build memorials—altars of stones—to remind them of miraculous events (Josh. 4:1–9). When God answers a prayer, or provides a miraculous intervention for your safety, make a memorial. Pick up a rock and place it on the mantle to remind you of when you almost fell from a cliff but God helped you grab onto a tree and be saved. Take home a seashell from the beach to remember that perfect evening when you walked along the shore, watched a beautiful sunset, and agreed with David that the heavens declare the glory of God. When you are feeling low, walk around the house and consider your personal stories of God's faithfulness as you look at your spiritual mementoes.

Warning signs

Through each of the steps mentioned, God will help you develop increased spiritual coping strength. But even so, it is important that you be very aware and respond to the warnings that signal you are nearing the end of your spiritual strength. These signals may include a lack of desire to fellowship, pray, or read the Bible. Other warning signs may be an inclination to give into temptation, a relaxing of your integrity, or rationalizing excuses for not doing what is right. You may feel as though God is far away and doesn't care about or for you.

If you are experiencing these symptoms, ask your heavenly Father to increase your faith—your shield against the fiery darts of wickedness (Eph. 6:16). Develop your spiritual strength. Don't be defeated.

Develop Mental Strength to Avoid Distress

The mind is an incredible thing. It is powerful. In fact, the Bible says that what you think determines what you are (Prov. 23:7). Too often we allow ourselves to get into destructive thinking habits. Paul reminds us to carefully watch what we think (2 Cor. 10:5; Phil. 4:7–9).

Usually it is not what happens that causes stress but what you tell yourself about what happens. If a friend fails to call you for a week, that would not necessarily be stressful. But if you tell yourself your friend must be angry with you, then you may become stressed. If someone drives around your car and darts into a parking space in front of you, that may not be stressful. But if you were headed for that parking space, then you will most likely experience stress reactivity.

Learn to develop thinking patterns that reduce your stress rather than increase it. Several years ago my husband and I were planning a trip to Egypt. We knew we would walk a lot in Egypt's very hot temperatures. A month before we were scheduled to leave, we drove to the grocery store. The only parking space we found was at the outer edge of a very large and crowded parking lot. I became a bit grumpy and started to complain. My husband said, "Come on, let's just pretend we're practicing for Egypt!"

My grumpiness faded. I laughed, caught his hand, and together we marched across the imagined desert sands of the parking lot. "Practicing for Egypt" has now become our password to remind us not to let destructive thoughts cause us unnecessary stress.

Steps to mental coping strength

• Clarify your beliefs.

If you expect yourself to be perfect all the time, you have a problem. According to the Bible, everyone falls short of perfection (Rom. 3:23; 1 John 1:10). If you expect everyone to like and approve of you, you will feel terrible rejection when you are criticized. Only God loves you unconditionally. He forgives you totally in Jesus—every time you make a mistake.

- Don't set unrealistic expectations.

When a project fails, do you feel like a personal failure? You aren't. Failure is simply discovering one wrong way. Failure is a signal to start over and try again.

What unrealistic expectations do you have for yourself and others? If your expectations are too high or unrealistic, you are setting yourself up to be constantly disappointed—a stressor. Your body will respond with stress reactivity. You will be ready to physically attack the person(s) who let you down. You may not actually hit or verbally lash out at that person, but you will probably at least be irritated or angry.

Do you believe that life should be fair?

Do you expect to always be rewarded for hard work?

Do you think you can please everyone?

Do you think wrongdoers ought to be swiftly punished?

Do you consider failure a disaster?

Do you think that everyone ought to be polite to one another?

Do you think that you are entitled to special treatment?

If so, you need to reassess the beliefs upon which you base your life. Decide which are realistic and which are unrealistic. Unrealistic beliefs will become stressors because they cannot be met. By changing your beliefs, you can reduce your stress reactivity and become more gentle in your relationships with others. You will be more understanding of differences in people (Phil. 4:5; Gal. 5:22–23).

- Don't expect life to be fair.

  Things won't always appear to be equitable.

- Don't expect people to always do what you think they ought to do.

  It doesn't make sense to get upset when others fail to behave nicely; fail to be open, honest, and caring; or fail to treat you with respect. Jesus said there would be thieves who come in the night to steal (Matt. 6:19–21). Instead of getting upset, ask the Lord to protect you and keep you from being a victim.

- Don't try to be a people pleaser.

- Don't assume the worst; assume the best.

  See what a difference it will make.

- Learn how things work.

    You may not like what you learn, but find out how things work. If you want to be promoted, find out how promotions are earned in your company. If you want to get a degree, find out what the specific requirements are and how you could fulfill them. Rather than hoping, discover what you can actually do. Christ will help you continue to do what is right.

- Read positive, uplifting books.

    Some books will inspire you. Some will inform you. Some will encourage you. Some will educate you. Read at least 30 minutes a day. If you fail to feed your mind, don't be surprised if your mind feeds you bad thoughts.

- Practice positive self talk.

    If you are like most people, you talk to yourself all the time. Do you talk to yourself in negative terms? When you make a mistake, do you tell yourself, "I'm so stupid"? When you fail, do you think, "I should have known better. Why can't I do anything right"? You wouldn't accept such criticism from anybody else. Why do you accept negativism from yourself?

    You may feel stupid when you do or say something foolish, but you are far from stupid. You do lots of things right, so don't call yourself incompetent when you botch something. We all have an infinite ability to learn and improve. Focus on the positive and use the "last time" as a teacher for the "next time." If you don't focus on how to do it better next time, you are doomed to repeat the past mistakes over and over again.

Solomon said that a soft answer turns away wrath (Prov. 15:1). This holds true not only as we deal with others but also when we talk to ourselves.

Warning signs

When you approach the end of your mental coping strength, you will become prone to mental distress. You may have a negative perspective. You may even have evil thoughts or thoughts of revenge against someone who has wronged you. You will be disappointed in people, in yourself, and in life. In extreme cases you may have neurotic thoughts or become paranoid. You may believe that everyone is out to harm you.

Take care of your mind. Let the peace of God keep your heart and mind (Phil. 4:7). Don't be distressed.

Develop Psychological Strength to Avoid Depression

Much of our psychological strength comes from

a strong sense of self-esteem. If you believe you can cope with whatever comes your way, you will. Even if circumstances are unpleasant, you will feel strong and unafraid. If you can experience fear without believing that it will conquer you, your ability to be courageous will surface. If you recognize that you are not required to be a pleaser of people but pleasing to God (Gal. 1:10), you are better prepared to face life from a strong psychological position.

Each of us is designed by God. We are wonderful creations (Ps. 139:13–17). We are God's handiwork, created to do good things (Eph. 2:10). Before the foundations of the world, God had in mind that we would become conformed to the image of Christ (Rom. 8:29). We are accepted in Christ by grace, just as we are (Eph. 1:6). God considered each one of us so valuable that He sacrificed His own Son, Jesus, to pay the price necessary to make us His own (1 Peter 1:18–19).

In view of these Scriptures, God considers us very valuable. We also ought to consider ourselves—and treat ourselves—as something of great value. If you would like to improve yourself in some way, you would be wise to begin working on it. Ask God for help. If there are impurities in your life, ask Jesus to eliminate them. If there are ways you might become better, ask for the Spirit's strength to strive for improvement.

People with an unhealthy self-esteem develop an "I can't" approach to life. They expect others to be rescuers, to be caretakers, to be protectors. In the process, the person with low self-esteem becomes even more dependent, weak, incompetent, and lazy.

Steps to psychological coping strength

- Assess yourself.

    Take an honest look at yourself and evaluate what you see. What kind of a friend, employee, supervisor, parent, son/daughter, mother/father, brother/sister, Christian, citizen, student/teacher, neighbor are you? List adjectives that describe you in these (and other) roles.

- Make a list of things you might do to improve yourself in each of these roles.

- Ask God for help. Develop an action plan for implementing an improvement program.

- Implement and monitor your action plan.

- Ask a friend how he/she sees you in each role.

- Surround yourself with positive, affirming Christian friends.

- Develop your skills in areas where you want to improve and excel.

Warning signs

Sometimes under stressful conditions you may discover your healthy self-esteem has deteriorated. You may begin to feel criticized, incapable, and unsure of yourself. You may feel afraid, hesitant, shy, intimidated, or depressed. Depression is sometimes defined as anger turned inward. Aiming anger at yourself indicates a low self-esteem. You may have failed to meet the high expectations you set for yourself. Whatever the cause, when your self-esteem is too low, ask the Spirit to remind you of what you are in Jesus—precious, valuable, and capable. Christ can help correct your self-esteem problem and enable you to cope with the stressors in life. Don't be depressed.

Develop Social Strength to Avoid Desertion

Ever feel you have been deserted by everyone who cares about you? Ever feel all alone? Most people experience these feelings at one time or another. They are not pleasant feelings. After God created Adam, He created Eve. God said it was not good for a person to be alone in the world (Gen. 2:18).

When your ability to cope diminishes, often good friends can help you recuperate and regain your strength. Therefore you will want to develop a strong social network. You undoubtedly have several casual acquaintances in your life. You may share an event with these people as you attend the same church or work together in the same company. Acquaintances provide a sense of belonging. You will also probably have several friends (15–20) in your life. You enjoy a variety of activities together: bowling, fishing, dining out, and so on. Friends provide enrichment, excitement, enjoyment, and encouragement in your life. You will also need two or three close friends in your life. A close friend, or buddy, shares what is really going on in your life—your struggles and your victories. In each of these groups of people (acquaintances, friends, and buddies), you will probably want to include men and women and have a balance between single and married, younger and older people.

This social structure can provide the social coping strength you need when you cannot cope alone. Paul said that none of us lives or dies alone (Rom. 14:8). We need a strong social network. We need to develop social coping strengths.

Steps to developing social coping strength

1. List your acquaintances.

    Make a list of the casual acquaintances in your life. If you can't list them by name, list them by group (e.g., church members, class members, club members, fellow employees).

2. List your friends and how each person adds to your life.

3. Make a list of your buddies and what things you feel comfortable sharing with each one.

4. Analyze your lists.

If you don't have two or three buddies, identify two or three people from your list of friends whom you would like to be your buddies. Plan how you might spend more time alone with each one. See if you can develop the close relationships you want. Remember that both people must want the closer relationship for it to work. If you don't have 15–20 friends, then identify people from your acquaintances with whom you would like to be friends and plan to spend time doing things together.

A second part of developing social strength involves sharpening your interpersonal skills so that your relationships and friendships will be constructive.

• Speak out.

It is not desirable to open your mouth every time you have a thought, but biting your tongue to keep from saying anything at all isn't healthy either. Somewhere between these two is an appropriate choice. Don't be afraid to share your opinions or ideas at appropriate times. Your idea may be good and may even lead to a better idea through discussion.

Remember the story of the feeding of the 5,000 in John 6:1–14? Andrew didn't know how to feed the people, but he did bring the small boy to Jesus and pointed out that the lad had some fish and bread. Jesus used what the boy had to feed everyone.

Perhaps you don't usually share your ideas because you don't want to look foolish, don't want to start an argument, don't want to be given additional responsibility based on your ideas, or don't want to be proven wrong. Consequently, you may have just kept quiet. But God doesn't want you to be a fearful person (2 Tim. 1:7). So speak out. Start with simple situations and practice until you feel comfortable speaking up. Then try a more difficult situation and still another.

• Learn to productively confront.

Most people experience difficulty confronting others. Confronting means bringing up negative and opposing ideas, not necessarily arguing. There are times when it is not only appropriate but necessary to confront. A child playing with matches is an obvious example. If not confronted, the child and others may be hurt. (See the story of the prophet Nathan and King David in 2 Sam. 12:1–7. Also see Jesus' conversation with the woman at the well in John 4:1–26.)

Confrontation often involves honestly talking out negative feelings. Without honesty, a relationship lacks true intimacy. Paul says that speaking the truth in love need not make enemies (Gal. 4:16; Eph. 4:15). Author John Powell reminds us, however, that kindness without honesty is phoney, but honesty without kindness is cruelty. When you confront, you must do it with kindness and love. Your goal must be to strengthen the relationship.

If you cannot talk to the person toward whom you have negative feelings, then find a good friend who will listen as you vent or express your feelings. A good friend will listen and still love you; listen and not necessarily give advice; listen and be understanding.

Are you harboring negative feelings you need to express? You are only hurting yourself and increasing your stress reactivity. The only way to get rid of negative feelings is to express them, release them, and forgive them.

Talk to God in prayer.

Write a letter.

Write in your journal.

Talk to the person involved.

Talk with a friend.

Talk with a counselor.

Walk on the beach and talk aloud to yourself.

Imagine the person you need to confront sitting in a chair facing you and carry on an imaginary conversation with that person.

- Ask for what you need.

    If you don't ask for what you need, you assume people will read your mind. By not voicing your needs, they may not be met, and resentment might build up. If your request is reasonable, approach the right person, ask without demanding, and allow the person the right to refuse your request. There is nothing wrong with asking for what you need.

    Paul voiced his needs to the Corinthians. He asked them to collect for the saints each week instead of waiting until he arrived (1 Cor. 16:1–3). Paul let the people know how he would like things done.

- Set reasonable limits.

    If it's difficult for you to set limits, people probably take advantage of you. Perhaps you believe genuine friends never say no to requests. Take a look at Jesus' life. Even our Lord refused some requests. Jesus refused to be made king and rescue the people from Roman rule (John 6:15). He refused to grant James and John a seat on either side of Him in heaven (Mark 10:35–40).

Say no to requests that unreasonably infringe upon your time, your goals, and your plans. At first, saying no may be hard, but you will soon develop confidence as you take the step in caring for yourself.

- Initiate contact

It can be intimidating to initiate that first contact or attempt to deepen a relationship from a friendship to a close friendship. You may fear rejection. If you truly want to develop your social strength, you must take the risk.

Zacchaeus wanted to see Jesus so badly that he climbed a tree in order to see over the crowds. A grown man risked being called foolish just to get a better glimpse as Jesus walked by. Jesus stopped beneath the tree and not only talked with Zacchaeus but went home with him for supper. Zacchaeus' life was changed forever (Luke 19:1–10). You'll never know what friendships await you unless you risk instead of holding back. Fear is one of life's biggest stressors.

- Give and receive compliments.

A poised person can give compliments without gushing and accept them without arrogance. Solomon reminds us that good words make us feel good. They are sweet to the soul and as precious as silver and gold (Prov. 12:25; 15:23; 16:24; 25:11). You can learn how to give and receive compliments graciously and gracefully.

Paul reminds us not to think of ourselves as more than we are. We need to honestly appraise ourselves. God gives each of us gifts and abilities. Recognize and appreciate these gifts and use them for the glory of God (Rom. 12:3–8).

- Express love and affection.

For some people, learning to express love and affection is difficult. Difficult or not, this is an important social skill.

Remember the woman who came to the dinner at Simon's house and cried over Jesus' feet, dried them with her hair, then anointed His feet with expensive ointment (Luke 7:36–50)? Jesus did not reject this woman's expressions of love, even though they were unusual. Jesus did not consider it unmanly to express love and affection. He demonstrated His love and affection to His disciples and those around Him. Jesus even commands us to love one another (John 13:34–35).

- Listen attentively.

     One of the more important skills necessary to develop relationships is the ability to listen attentively and empathetically without judging and without interrupting. James would agree. He said we ought to be quick to listen, and slow to speak (James 1:19).

If you have problems with interpersonal skills, social problems probably provide major stressors in your life. You may want to work to improve these skills so that you can eliminate these stressors and reduce your stress reactivity. For additional assistance in this area you may want to read *Pleasing You Is Destroying Me* by Bobbie Reed (WORD, 1992).

Warning signs

If, when you go to parties or functions, you always arrive late, stand by yourself, and leave early; if you have no one to call when you feel lonely; if you can't find someone to share your two-for-one coupon for dinner; and if you can't identify friends or buddies in your life, you probably need to focus attention on your social network. Ask the Spirit to help you develop your social coping strength. Don't be deserted.

More benefits

One of the interesting side benefits of developing your coping strengths is that you often eliminate some of the stressors and relieve your stress reactivity. We will look at a more intentional approach to these two aspects in the next chapters.

3
❡ Eliminate Some Stressors

Meet the Johnsons.

Bill Johnson is 39 years old and works as a supervisor in the marketing department at Metrocom Systems. Because of the slowed economy there is pressure in the company to increase sales. There has also been talk about cutting staff and reorganizing the company's management structure. Recently the company upgraded their computer system, and everyone had to learn the new system. Bill's car has been acting up, and he hasn't decided whether to buy a new one or have the old one repaired. Because of some unexpected bills (braces for his daughter and a new wardrobe for his son who grew five inches over the summer), the family budget is tight and balances due on the credit cards are high. Bill was asked to serve as coordinator for an upcoming mission conference at church and is seriously considering the request. Lately Bill can't sleep. He often wakes up in the middle of the night and thinks about his problems. He gets up in the mornings feeling tired. Bill takes more headache tablets lately. His stress reactivity has become noticeable.

Joanne Johnson, Bill's wife, is 37 and works as an X-ray technician at a local clinic. She feels guilty about not being home when her children come home from school (Tracy is 12 and David is 17) but realizes that the family could not get along without her salary. Joanne is being promoted to supervising X-ray technician and will supervise three X-ray technicians with whom she has worked for the last three years. She is apprehensive about the change in relationships but is excited about the promotion. Joanne's best friend moved to Japan last month and will be gone for two years. Joanne, always struggling with her weight, started a new diet. She also signed up for an aerobics class on Tuesdays and Thursdays. These classes will cause a bit of juggling with her schedule because she takes David to various after-school activities and Tracy to the orthodontist. The many changes in Joanne's life have caused her to experience a degree of stress reactivity. The family notices that she is more irritable, more easily upset, and nervous.

Tracy started junior high school this year. Because she is in a special arts program, Tracy goes to a different school than most of her friends from sixth grade. The new school is a distance from home so she must get up a half hour earlier to arrive on time. Some of Tracy's classmates have suggested she experiment with drugs. Although Tracy has consistently refused to do so, she feels significant peer pressure to do what "everyone else is doing." Tracy is also self-conscious about her new braces. Tracy has become a little withdrawn. She spends more time alone in her room after school and appears to be somewhat depressed. She also experiences stress reactivity.

David just got his first car. In order to pay for gas and insurance, he works at a fast-food restaurant on weekends and some evenings. David continues to send for literature from various colleges to help him decide where he will go in the fall. David's grandpa wants him to go to his alma mater. Bill would like David to go to the college he attended. Joanne prefers the community college so David could live at home for a few more years. David would like to attend a big college back East, but unless he gets a scholarship, he knows he can't afford that. Last week David broke off his three-year relationship with his girlfriend. Although David is pretty sure breaking up was the right decision, he misses her and sometimes is tempted to slip back into the comfortable relationship—especially when she calls, crying about their breakup. David feels everyone is pushing or pulling him, and all in different directions. David's temper is on a short fuse, and lately he says things in anger that he later regrets. David is stressed.

The Johnsons are a typical American family. Each of the family members experiences stressors and stress reactivity.

Identify the Stressors

When Bill Johnson became aware of his stress reactivity (frequent headaches and periodic sleep loss), he decided to take a look at his life and attempt to reduce the stressors. Bill listed the major stressors he could identify.

Changes

- Fear of layoff
- Fear of company restructuring

Challenges

- Pressure to increase company sales
- Need to learn the new computer system
- Decision concerning the car
- Opportunity to serve as mission conference coordinator
- Work brought home every evening and not finished
- Need to clean the garage (on his list of things to do six weeks ago)
- Guilt about not spending quality time with the family

Conflicts

- Uncertainty about what his boss really thinks of his work
- Financial concerns
- Traffic problems on the way to work

- Need to talk to neighbor about not borrowing the lawn mower without permission (planned to do this for several months)

- Hating to come home—always bombarded as soon as he walks into the house (kids wanting things, wife asking for assistance with supper preparations)

- Serving as a telephone answering service for his children

- Not being able to eat dinner or watch a television show without the telephone ringing several times

Bill stopped writing and looked at his list in disbelief. He hadn't realized there were so many things acting as stressors in his life on an ongoing basis. Added to the listed items were the confrontations on the job, minor arguments with Joanne and the children, and daily frustrations. Bill suddenly recognized that he needed to take some action to reduce the stressors in his life.

It is impossible to eliminate all, or even most, of the stressors in life. But you can make some changes that will reduce stressors and improve your well-being. Here are some things Bill decided to do.

Bill admitted to himself that one of the stressors in his life was feeling all alone in his responsibility for the family. Although he considered Joanne his partner, Bill still believed the ultimate responsibility for decisions belonged to him. That pressure weighed heavily on him.

After completing his assessment (listing changes, challenges, and conflicts), Bill could see that he had become so busy he had failed to maintain a strong personal relationship with God. He had failed in his discipline to spend at least 20 minutes a day alone, communicating with God. In order to develop his spiritual strength, Bill designed an aggressive plan. He would start his day by reading the Bible.

Bill considered several alternatives but decided to start reading through the New Testament by reading at least three chapters a day. Other alternatives might include using a devotional book or one of the programs for Bible reading developed by various sources.

Bill made a conscious decision to give priority to prayer. Before and after reading the Bible, Bill would pray that God would help him draw from that Scripture the lessons he would need for that day. He would ask for God's input into his priorities and for a proper attitude and perspective on the events of the day. In essence, Bill invited God to be his partner in day-to-day decisions.

Are there areas of your life where you are trying to go it alone? Remember that Jesus promised to be with you always (Matt. 28:20). We need not function in our own strength. Remember! With Christ you can do all things (Phil. 4:13.)

Eliminate as Many Stressors as Possible.

As Bill looked at his list, he realized that he could take charge. He could eliminate some of the stressors.

- Start early.

Bill knew he had to leave home at 7:20 each morning to get to work by 8:00. He almost always arrived at work on time, but whenever the traffic slowed on the freeway, Bill became anxious that he might be late for work. Bill decided he could eliminate that stressor by leaving for work at 7:00 and having his devotions in the car in the parking lot. He was spending the same amount of time commuting and having personal devotions, but by scheduling that time differently, he eliminated several stressors. In addition, by arriving earlier, Bill usually found a parking space close to the building's entrance (eliminating a stressor that had not even been on his original list).

Are there ways you can rearrange your schedule to better use the available time and eliminate stressors? Paul says in Ephesians 5:15–16 to be wise and make the most of our time.

- Find out about changes at work.

Instead of fearing the changes and pressures at work, Bill decided to have a frank discussion with his boss. Bill explained that he felt a bit anxious about the possible company changes. He asked his boss for input.

Bill's boss couldn't give Bill all the details about upcoming changes, but he did reassure Bill that his work was outstanding. He reassured Bill there was no need to worry about a layoff. Together Bill and his boss discussed the need for increased success in marketing the company's products. They came up with several possible approaches. That stressor had become less stressful.

Bill also realized that by spending only a few minutes here and there to learn the new computer system, he had not made much progress. He went to the training manager and asked about available options for learning the new system. Bill learned an on-screen tutorial program could be installed on his computer. The tutorial could also be checked out and taken home, and a two-day class was also planned. Bill opted for the class. In two short days, he became proficient with the program, and another big hurdle in his life was cleared.

Living with vague concerns about what may or may not happen allows stressors to control your life. Instead, see what you can find out

about the possibilities. You may not learn everything you want to know, but searching for
answers is more healthy and productive than
worrying. The more you learn about the possibilities, the easier it will be to plan for the even-
tualities. Study how things work, and apply
yourself so you can be a good student, pleasing
to God (2 Tim. 2:15).

- Keep lists of things to do.

*One source of arguments between Joanne and
Bill was Bill's forgetfulness. Bill didn't mean to forget, but with so many other things on his mind, he
just couldn't keep everything straight. Bill decided to
become a "make a list" person.*

*Bill started at work. Each night before coming
home, he would list the telephone calls to make the
next day, people to see, and meetings. He noticed that
within days his efficiency increased. The list was easy
to compose at the end of the work day because the
things to list were uppermost in his mind after working with the related issues all day.*

*Bill became more dependable at home. He listed
household repairs Joanne wanted done. He took a list
to the store. He noted important dates—his son's
football games, his daughter's piano recital. In the
past, Bill forgot such events and felt very guilty and
angry with himself.*

When depending on his memory, Bill found all the things to be done were stressors. When Bill made a checklist of things to do, it eliminated his worry about forgetting and also gave him a record of what he had accomplished.

Why waste your memory trying to remember everything you need to do? Make lists. Get organized. Plan your schedule. When you make a list, you get a realistic picture of just how much you can commit to doing. Don't be subject to ridicule or rejection because you didn't count the cost or can't live up to your grandiose plans to do it all (Luke 14:28–30).

- Learn to say no.

When the pastor called Bill to get his answer about coordinating the mission conference, Bill said yes. He knew he didn't have time for the extra work, but Bill didn't feel comfortable saying no to such a worthwhile endeavor. In retrospect Bill decided he needed to learn to say no more often to demands or requests that would become stressors in his life.

To practice, Bill looked at some of the commitments in his life where he had the option to say no. He decided to resign as secretary/scorekeeper for the bowling league. He didn't try out for the lead in the community play. Bill asked one of the other fathers to drive part of the time to the high school football games. These were small steps, but for Bill they were profitable. He stopped volunteering beyond his ability to comfortably fulfill obligations.

Do you have a problem saying no? Paul says in Colossians 4:4–6 that we must be careful when we respond to people. We need to carefully consider our time and our commitments. Sometimes the response needs to be no.

- Don't be a slave to the telephone.

Just when Bill sits down in the evenings to talk with Joanne, the telephone rings. Often it's a caller for one of the children. "I feel like an answering service!" Bill complained one evening to Joanne. "We never get to talk without interruptions."

There was a simple solution. Bill invested in a telephone answering system. It allowed Bill to answer the telephone if he was free or ignore it if he didn't want to be interrupted. Other parents have installed separate telephone lines (with answering machines) for the children. The system is placed in a downstairs family room or other area where the sound of ringing is no longer an interruption.

Are there machines that can assist you in reducing some of the stressors in your life? Investigate them. The initial cost may seem high, but with careful budgeting, you may be able to afford something that will significantly improve the quality of your life by reducing stress.

- Develop a budget plan.

Even though bankruptcy was not a threat, Bill and Joanne's financial situation was a stressor to both of them. Bill knew he must decide what to do about his car. Together they decided to review their finances and their financial decision making process. They developed a workable budget plan. Taking these steps helped Bill and Joanne make a decision about the car.

Living beyond your financial resources can be a terrific strain and stressor. Paul says the ideal is not to owe anyone anything (Rom. 13:8). In today's world it seems almost impossible not to have debts (e.g., home mortgage, car payments). If we live too close to our limits, then the fear of not being able to pay the bills can become a strong stressor. A realistic financial plan can alleviate this stressor.

- Stop procrastinating.

Bill opened his eyes one Saturday morning and groaned. He knew there were several things he ought to do, but he didn't want to tackle any of them. He didn't have the energy. Then Bill decided to make this Saturday a "cleanup day." He would spend the day doing all the little things that had been on his list forever.

Bill cleaned the garage, talked to his neighbor

about borrowing the lawn mower, had the car tuned up, pruned the bushes, wrote the checks for the bills, dropped off his clothes at the cleaners, and repaired the broken shelf in the linen closet. He replaced the light bulb in the high ceiling fixture (it had been out for two months). Then Bill finished up by taking the bags of aluminum cans to the recycling center— clearing lots of room in the garage. Bill finished his chores by 4:00 and decided to take the family out to dinner to celebrate. Bill felt energized because of the lack of pressure. He felt satisfied and proud because he completed his list of little things to do.

Procrastination is a stressor because it allows you to build up a long list of things you haven't done. These nag you and weigh on your mind. They keep you from enjoying planned relaxation or recreation. Take a look at your list. Cross off the tasks you won't ever do. Getting the rest taken care of will eliminate a lot of stressors in your life.

Solomon invites us to consider the ant. It does not give in to laziness, rather it takes care of business. The ant gathers food when it is time to gather food. It does what needs doing, in a timely way (Prov. 6:6–8).

• Set aside time for self and family.

The minute Bill came home from work, he felt

bombarded by requests and demands. He wasn't ready to face the family. He needed to spend a few minutes alone to make the transition from work to home. Bill asked the family to give him the first 30 minutes after he returned home to be by himself. After that time, he promised to be available to the family. They agreed.

Some days Bill took a shower. Other days he would read the paper, watch the news, take a nap, finish up his paperwork from the office, read the mail, sit on the patio and drink a cup of coffee, walk around the block, make a few telephone calls, or work in the garage on his current carpentry project. Knowing that he had 30 minutes all to himself was a wonderful relief. He could get things done, take care of himself, retreat from demands, and relax.

For about the next 30 minutes, Bill dealt with family issues. He found he actually listened better to the children's stories about school, made better decisions about their requests, and was more attentive to Joanne. Instead of feeling bombarded and wanting to retreat, Bill was ready to give to his family.

Other families have decided to set aside a family night. Nothing is allowed to infringe upon this special family time. Family members may run in different directions all the other days of the week, but on that one night, they all come together. They work together on projects, talk, play, or engage in an activity that everyone enjoys. Quality time with the family is important because parents need this time to teach children, love them, and encourage them in their spiritual journeys as well as encourage their personal maturity (Prov. 22:6; Eph. 6:4).

• Reduce noise.

Bill decided to eliminate some of the noise in his life. Because the laundry room was just off the family room, the noise of doing the wash was a major interruption. After discussion with Joanne, they agreed to move the washer and dryer into the garage where the noise could not be heard inside the house.

The sound of the children's stereos, however muted, could be heard in the family room also. Bill invested in headphones for each of the children. They were pleased because they could listen to their music as loudly as they wished, and the beat of the drums and guitars no longer filtered into the family room.

Although they loaded the dishwasher immediately after supper, Joanne and Bill decided not to run it until they went upstairs to bed. This eliminated the noise of that appliance too.

Bill and Joanne further decided to turn on the television only when they watched a specific program. In the past, the TV played continually, whether or not anyone was watching. The quiet was a little hard to get used to, but soon Bill and Joanne began to enjoy it.

Loud or continuous noise can be a significant stressor. Other families have been inventive in eliminating noise from their lives. They have learned to enjoy the soothing quiet. Isaiah talked of finding peace and a quiet resting place (Is. 32:17–18). Paul talked to the church at Thessalonica about the virtue of quiet (1 Thess. 4:11–12).

- Check out pain.

As Bill thought about his stressors, he realized that the almost-constant pain in his knee for the past three weeks created a stress reactivity. He dismissed the pain as "probably arthritis" or would comment that he must be getting old, but he didn't take any steps to check on or eliminate the pain. When Bill went to his doctor, he recommended the appropriate treatment, and after a period of time, Bill's pain went away.

Do you experience pain that may need medical attention? Take care of it soon. Don't allow these stressors to affect your life. Jesus was often approached by people who needed physical healing. Jesus recognized their needs. He healed the lepers, the palsied, those with fevers, and many others. Today, God has empowered doctors with incredible medical knowledge that can be useful in healing our bodies and reducing stressful pain.

- Turn from sin.

After Bill eliminated or reduced most of the stressors over which he had some control, he realized one stressor wasn't listed. Bill had had a heated argument with a friend. He said very hurtful things and hadn't spoken to his friend in more than a month. Each time Bill tried to pray, the Holy Spirit would remind him of the broken relationship. He reminded Bill that God's standard required making peace with one's brother (Matt. 5:23–24). Bill stubbornly resisted because he had been hurt by his friend's attitude and felt bitter toward his friend. One day Bill's daily Bible reading included Ephesians 4:29–32. Bill knew he could no longer resist. He had to forgive—had to put aside the malice and bitterness in his own heart. Bill called his friend, and both agreed to meet. They worked through their mutual pain to reestablish the relationship.

Sin is a major stressor because it puts a barrier between ourselves and God (Ps. 66:18; John 9:31; 1 John 1:7). Ask the Spirit to show you areas in your life where sin exists. God can remove this stressor from your life.

After a few weeks, Bill was surprised how less stressful his life felt. His headaches went away, he was more patient with the family, and more productive at work. Follow Bill's example. Consider the stressors in your own life. Review your list and examine each one carefully. You will be surprised how a little bit of creativity can help eliminate many stressors. You will feel better, and you will also become more productive.

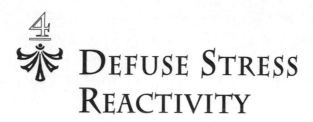

DEFUSE STRESS REACTIVITY

"I'm so cranky lately," Joanne admitted to her friend, *Sally. "I don't like the person I've become. I don't know what to do. I feel as if I'm hanging on by my fingernails and one of them is about to break."*

"Sounds as if you are under a lot of stress," Sally responded. *"Why don't you sign up for that stress class they are offering next week at work? I took it and I learned a lot."*

Joanne considered Sally's suggestion and decided to take the class. She needed to do something.

Taking the class turned out to be a wonderful suggestion. Joanne learned that she could actually learn to control her response to stressors and thus reduce her stress reactivity. Here are some of the things Joanne began to practice.

Use Up Excess Energy

Whenever you have been exposed to a significant stressor or to accumulated stressors, your body gears up its stress reactivity response. It infuses your systems with excess energy. As we have already indicated in previous chapters, when excess energy is generated, it causes the body to perpetuate the resistance stage of the stress response until the energy is used up. It is necessary, therefore, to use up that extra energy as soon as possible.

Physical work is a great way to drain off excess energy. Clean out the garage, mow the lawn, weed the garden, rearrange the closets, do your spring cleaning, paint the house (or at least a room), build something, or wash the car.

Try physically demanding recreational activity, such as fishing, hiking, swimming, canoeing, skiing, bicycling, running, jogging, or bowling. Play tennis, racquetball, basketball, football, softball, or baseball. Consider strenuous physical exercise such as aerobics, mat exercises, or weight lifting.

When you use up the excess energy, your body returns to normal functioning. The stress reactivity response stops. Another benefit is the concentration on the physical activity gives your mind a rest from thinking about the stressor.

Take Control

Often when you are under stress, you feel as if someone else is in control of your life. One solution is to take control in as many ways as you can.

Check your schedule. Are there commitments

you can change, postpone, delegate, or cancel without letting someone down? If so, do it. Are there things you need to tackle so they stop hanging over your head? Do them.

If someone barges into your office, starts to yell, and accuses you of something, you will probably experience a stress response. The same reaction can happen if someone verbally attacks you over the telephone. One way to take charge is offer to listen and work at resolving the issues in just a few minutes. Tell the intruder that you will meet him/her in 10 minutes to continue the discussion. Tell the telephone caller that you will pull the correspondence or file and call back in 10 minutes.

Use the 10 minutes to physically relax, take a short walk, get a drink of water, and prepare yourself mentally. Then meet the other person or return the telephone call. You will be surprised at the difference in your physical response. When you go to someone else's office, you are the initiator, not the victim. When you return the telephone call, you are the initiator, not the one under attack. Even if the person continues to attack, you are more in control than you were when they intruded into your space.

Another technique that helps you take control is to identify fears that are stressing you. If you are afraid that something might happen (layoffs, rejections, failed investments, inability to meet obligations, or undesirable assignments), don't sit and wait and wonder. Instead, find out if there is a basis for your fears. Make contingency plans that will cover you in case your worst fears come true. That way, you are better prepared and stress is lessened.

Jesus told a parable of five wise virgins. The young women didn't know what time the bridegroom would return, but they made plans and were ready. When the bridegroom eventually returned, there was no stress for the wise virgins. However, the foolish and unprepared virgins became very stressed because they had made no plans (Matt. 25:1–13).

If you feel as if you are not in control, look for things you can do to take charge of what is happening in your life. Don't worry. Plan.

Use Problem Solving Skills

Take steps to resolve your specific problems. Don't allow someone else's problems to keep you awake, especially if the other person is not worried or concerned. Research the problem issue and identify core issues. Then consider alternatives for resolving the problem. Select the option that seems most promising, and implement that solution. Check the results. If the issue is resolved, so is your stress problem in this case.

In problem solving, it is important to make decisions and then let them go. Don't spend the hours or days after making a decision second guessing your actions. Most of the time there is not just one right solution or one clear answer. If there were, problem solving would be easy. Therefore, you simply do the necessary research, make the best decision possible with the information you have, and work with your solution.

Find the Humor

One of the best tools in your stress reducing kit is your sense of humor. Whenever possible, try to find a humorous angle to your stressful situation. Consider what a great story the situation will make for you to use in entertaining your friends. Try to develop an ability to see the lighter side of situations when you are right in the middle of them.

I remember once I flew to another state to speak at an evening banquet. Because the flight took only a little over an hour, I left in the middle of the afternoon, dressed very casually for traveling. When I arrived at the airport, I found a nightmare of cancelled flights, upset people, and harried airline agents. My flight was delayed, as was the flight ahead of it. My plane was scheduled too late to get me to the banquet, so I asked if I could catch the flight just leaving. The agent looked out the window at the small plane and nodded, encouraging me to hurry.

Just then I saw my suitcase on a baggage cart

outside the door. Taking a chance, I asked if it would be possible to retrieve my suitcase. The agent looked at me with incredulity. Even though all he said was no, he managed to convey what he was really thinking. He had already helped me make an earlier flight, how could I possibly expect to also have my suitcase? I shrugged my shoulders and said, "Oh, well! I guess I'll just have to speak at the banquet dressed as I am."

Suddenly the agent looked up, gave me the once over, noted my mismatched slacks and t-shirt, my lack of makeup, and dashed out of the door for my suitcase. I didn't stop laughing until well after the plane had taken off.

Get Away

Getting away to rest, relax, and recharge your batteries can be an effective antidote for depletion of energy caused by too much stress. Your "getting away" could include a 20-minute mental vacation or a month-long European vacation. You may wish to go away with a friend or by yourself. But don't forget to plan times to get away from it all.

Ways to escape include: taking a vacation, going for a drive, sleeping, taking a break, closing your office door for an hour, call forwarding your telephone, or letting the answering machine or voice mail screen your telephone calls. You can listen to music, read, meditate on Scripture, pray, watch television or a movie, daydream. You may want to take a warm bath, sit in the jacuzzi, go to your bedroom and close the door, or check into a motel room and not let anyone know where you are (within reason, don't worry your family). A trip to the beach or the mountains can provide the getaway you need too.

Practice Acceptance and Forgiveness

If you experience unresolvable difficulties within the family, with friends, or at work, they will continue to be stressful for you. There are two main ways to reduce your stress in this area. First, learn to accept people for who they are and where they are in their developmental journeys rather than who or where you wish they were.

Perhaps you work for a man who is driving you crazy. You think your boss ought to be nicer, kinder, more reasonable, or more decisive. Ask the Holy Spirit to help you accept him the way he is. If you can't work with him the way he is, then take steps to change jobs.

Perhaps you wish your spouse was different. Accept that person the way he/she is. You can discuss your desire for change with your spouse, but be aware that insisting on change rarely works. Changes made under pressure seldom last long.

Perhaps you wish you were more than or better

than you are. Accept your limitations. Begin working to become more like your desired ideal. But start with self acceptance. God accepts us, by grace, as we are, even though we presently fall short of the divine plan (Rom. 3:23; Eph. 2:8–9).

The second step is to forgive what you can't accept. When you have been hurt, disappointed, let down, betrayed, rejected, or criticized, the only way to let go of the pain is to forgive. Forgiveness doesn't let the other person off the hook, it lets you off the hook. Forgiveness doesn't mean the other person was right, or that in eternal terms there won't be a penalty, it just means that you no longer pay the painful penalty for what someone else has done.

We as Christians are commanded to be kind to one another and tenderhearted, to forgive one another as God, for Christ's sake, forgave us (Eph. 4:32).

When the Spirit helps you accept people and hurts, your stress reactivity can be reduced and your life can return to normal functioning.

Pamper Yourself

Sometimes it is helpful to pamper yourself as a way of relieving stress. Get a massage, have your hair styled, allow yourself to cry, scream (in a safe place, of course), punch out an imaginary enemy by using a bat and a pillow, dine out, laugh (rent a funny video), entertain, talk with a friend/spouse, go shopping (be sure your budget can afford what you buy), cook your favorite meal, have fun doing your favorite things, listen to your favorite music.

In the midst of His busy life, Jesus took time to go eat with His friends Mary, Martha, and Lazarus. He napped in the boat as the disciples rowed across the sea. It's okay for you to pamper yourself once in a while as long as you don't cultivate a selfish lifestyle and always insist on taking care of your own needs first.

Get Assistance

When you have difficulty thinking things through clearly, call a friend. When you need information, seek it out. When your prayers don't seem to go further than the ceiling, call fellow Christians and ask for prayer.

Sometimes, you may find it helpful to seek professional counseling to assist you through a difficult problem or period in your life. Don't be afraid to tap into this resource. Often another person can see your problem more clearly because you are so emotionally involved. Also, trained professionals can provide the assistance you need to help you return to normal functioning as soon as you work through your immediate problems/issues.

Taking steps to specifically reduce your stress reactivity produces great benefits. You will feel better, be able to think more clearly, and you will be more effective and productive in your relationships and on your job.

Part II: Cope with Stress in the Family

5

LIVE WITHIN YOUR BUDGET

One night during dinner, David brought up the family vacation. Everyone expressed different preferences and ideas. The costs of various options came up. Some of the ideas sounded great but were beyond the vacation budget the Johnsons could afford. So the discussion switched to the subject of money. The discussion was so important that the family decided to leave the dishes and adjourn to the family room so they could really get into the subject.

Problem Attitudes about Money

As they talked, the Johnsons discovered nonproductive attitudes about money. Do any of these ideas sound familiar?

- I use money to get even with others.

    Try communicating, confronting, and forgiving instead (see Matt. 5:23–25; Mark 11:25–26).

- I consider tithing to be living "under the law."

    Everything we have belongs to God (see

John 15:5; James 1:17; 1 Cor. 6:19–20; 2 Cor. 9:6–8).

- I use money to reward myself. If I achieve a goal, I give myself an expensive gift even if I can't afford it.

  The quality of your life does not depend on the number of possessions you have (see Luke 12:15).

- I like to give expensive gifts regardless of my budget. It's how I show love.

  You can't buy love. In order to be loved, you must love, not give gifts.

- It's my money. I earn it. I have a right to spend it and don't have to save for a rainy day. If an emergency occurs, I'll just borrow money.

  There's no "if" about it. Emergencies will occur. You need to prepare for them. Don't borrow money unless you absolutely must (Rom. 13:8).

- My spending habits are no one's business but my own.

  As a member of a family, spending habits are important not only to the individual involved but also to the entire family who may have to bear the consequences of a lack of funds. What hurts one member, hurts another (1 Cor. 12:26).

There are many other destructive attitudes people may have toward money, but these are some of the more common.

God's Plan for Our Money

There are three main reasons God allows us to have money: to honor Him and provide for God's work; to provide for ourselves and our families; and to provide for others in need.

Giving to God is both a responsibility and a privilege. When the Israelites failed to give to God, they were called "robbers" (Mal. 3:8). When you put God first with your money, you acknowledge His divine ownership of you and all that you have.

God has also given us the responsibility of providing for our families. We pay the bills, curtail unnecessary spending, save for emergencies and large expenditures, and provide shelter, clothing, food, education, and other necessities of life. Paul took a tough stand when he taught this principle. He stated that people who did not provide for their own had denied the faith and were worse than infidels (1 Tim. 5:8).

We also serve God and others as we provide for those in need. John wrote that if we have extra resources, see a brother in need, and do not help, we do not have the love of God dwelling in us (1 John 3:17–18).

A Good Plan

After discussing attitudes about money and God's purposes for giving us money, the Johnsons talked about how they ought to view their resources and use them wisely. They decided to follow principles based on God's Word.

- Put God first.

  Each member of the family planned to give God 10% of their income/allowance as a way to honor God.

- Avoid borrowing whenever possible.

  The family planned a way to pay off all current bills, except the house and the car. They agreed to buy with cash in the future. The family resolved that if they didn't have enough money saved to buy something, they would defer the purchase (Prov. 22:7).

- Make payments on time.

  The Johnsons decided to pay on time, no matter what else had to be sacrificed (Prov. 28:22). They determined not to get behind on their payments.

- Prepare for the future.

  Bill and Joanne looked into retirement options, put aside college money for the children (the children also planned to contribute), and saved for vacations and emergencies (Gen. 41:46–49, 53–57; Prov. 6:6–11; Luke 19:23).

- Don't buy just to keep up with the neighbors.

    The family set three rules for spending. If you don't need it, don't buy it. If you can't afford it, don't buy it. If you can get along without it, don't buy it (Luke 12:15).

- Wait for sales.

    When family members wanted something, they would put the item on a list of "want to haves." They would wait until they could find a bargain or a sale before making the purchase.

- Spend money to the glory of God.

    The Johnsons decided they would look at spending money as a way of bringing glory to God—not just as a way of acquiring things, paying bills, or rewarding themselves (1 Cor. 10:31).

Develop a Budget Plan

The next thing the Johnsons did was develop a realistic budget and financial plan. The plan included ways to get out of debt, ways to prepare for the future, and ways to implement the principles they had agreed to let govern their financial life as a family. When unexpected expenditures came up, they decided they would meet as a family and see if there were ways they could pull together, sacrifice together, and make the necessary payment. Bill and Joanne found the children very cooperative as they became a part of the planning committee and the decision making committee for the family budget.

Is Your Budget a Stressor?

Evaluate your spending habits. Take a close look at your attitudes about money. Review your budget plan. Is money a stressor because you aren't able to do all that you want to do with your income? Enlist the family's help to study your financial picture.

List the *changes* that have occurred in the last 12 months. Have you purchased a new car or home, run up the credit accounts, or had emergency medical expenses? Have you received unexpected income, been given a raise, or inherited money? Take these into consideration when developing a financial plan.

List the *challenges* (demands or pressures) to your budget. Are you overdue on paying some bills? Are there anticipated purchases that may challenge adherence to the budget plan?

List the *conflicts* that involve your finances. Are there competing priorities, needs, wants, and ideas about how the money should be spent? Are there conflicting attitudes within the family? How can these be productively resolved?

Once you identify these three types of stressors to your financial plan, you are ready to resolve issues, reduce stressors, and relieve your stress response.

Debt is a stressor. Unexpected expenses that push the limit of your resources cause stress. A lack of sufficient, available savings for emergencies is a stressor. Take control. Commit your spending patterns to God and you will reduce these stressors. Get started today. You'll be thrilled to see what a difference it makes.

6

DEAL WITH OCCUPATIONAL ISSUES

Bill and Joanne have already identified and dealt with the stressors at their jobs. However, related stressors might be causing you distress. See if you can identify with any of these stressors. You may want to take the actions suggested to eliminate them or to reduce your stress reactivity.

Job Stressors

- Too much to do.

    It's better to be busy at work than to have too little to do, but there is a limit to what can be accomplished. Do you work additional hours and still not finish the work on your desk? What can you do?

    Learn to delegate. Moses had to learn this lesson from his father-in-law, Jethro (Ex. 18:13–26).

    Learn to use your time effectively. If you allow interruptions to throw you off schedule, or if you plan an unrealistic schedule, you need to reevaluate. If you fail to group tasks that can be handled together, you may be wasting valuable time.

Set priorities. Can some of the things you are doing wait until later? Are some even necessary?

- Too little to do.

If you have too little to do, the work day will seem very long and you will be bored. This can result in stress. If this is your problem, you can:

Let your supervisor know that you are available for extra assignments.

Take advantage of training opportunities and expand your knowledge of the computer systems, the budget process, or any other phase of your company. In this way you will increase your value to the company and prepare yourself for additional responsibilities.

Help out your co-workers with their assignments. Perhaps in the future if your work picks up, they may be able to reciprocate. Even if they don't help you later, you will have learned more about their assignments and once again increase your value to the company.

Look around and see if there are systems that

could use improvement or streamlining. Put on your thinking cap and come up with suggestions.

- Unsure of your responsibilities.

Sometimes a supervisor will give you an assignment or put you into a new role but be vague about your responsibilities. This can cause stress because you won't know if you are fulfilling your supervisor's expectations. Also, if your new role puts you in a different relationship with co-workers, the lines of responsibility and authority need to be carefully delineated. If this is a problem, you can:

Meet with your supervisor and clarify expectations.

Ask for a session with your colleagues to discuss your new role.

Ask your supervisor if you are meeting your job responsibilities and what areas need improvement.

Keep the lines of communication open. Do not be afraid to approach your supervisor and ask for information.

- Too much discomfort.

Each new role or responsibility may feel uncomfortable to you at first, but with continued practice, you will find that your comfort level has expanded. Still, there may be some assignments that just aren't for you. If you cannot reconcile yourself to your new responsibilities, you may need to request a different assignment.

Sometimes you are told to handle a situation one way and you feel very strongly that you need to handle it another way. Speak up. Remember David? He had decided to go and fight Goliath. King Saul outfitted David in a suit of armor, but David felt too uncomfortable. He told Saul about his discomfort, and then David took another approach. God honored his stance, and David killed Goliath with a sling and a rock (1 Sam. 17:31–49).

• Too much comfort.

Perhaps you have worked at your job so long, and are so good at it, that the job no longer holds a challenge for you. Boredom at work is stressful. If this describes you, you may need to:

Pursue a promotion or at least a job rotation. This will force you to learn new skills and develop a different level of knowledge.

Look around and find something you do not know how to do within the company. Take steps to be trained in that area. Increase your value to the company and increase your chances for promotion in this way.

In the meantime, enroll in college classes. Earn a degree. Take up a new sport or hobby.

- Too much competition.

In some companies, competition is so strongly encouraged it becomes destructive. Sales persons competing with one another can increase sales, but managers competing with one another for status and resources can become secretive, selfish with information, and manipulative. When this type of atmosphere exists, you are bound to experience stress. You can:

Encourage all staff members to remember they are on the same team. Ask your supervisor to hold some team-building sessions.

Be open with your information and cooperative with your peers even if they don't reciprocate.

Point out the destructiveness of unhealthy competition.

Don't use comparisons with others in your reports and conversations.

In extreme cases, if you cannot resolve the matter, you may consider other employment.

- Too much change.

Your company may be one in which change is constant. Priorities change hourly. Policies are adapted to each new situation. This can be exciting and productive—depending on the type of business involved. But in most companies, this degree of flexibility is confusing for staff and creates stress and discomfort. If you are in a situation like this you can:

Discuss your observations with your supervisor. See if some basic policies and procedures can be established to provide stability for the organization.

Determine if the changes are because of a lack of written procedures. If this is the case, offer to draft necessary written procedures for your supervisor.

If the changes in priorities and deadlines occur because there is a lack of planning, suggest or initiate a strategic planning process in which you look far enough ahead to set appropriate priorities and deadlines.

- No change at all.

There are jobs where no new ideas are considered. The motto of these companies is "If it isn't broken, don't fix it." They refuse to consider flexible work hours, child care centers, job rotations, or reorganizations. If you are a person who sees the possibilities that could assist your company, and your company refuses to change, you may become stressed and frustrated. You can:

Suggest a few small changes that hold potential

for increasing profits or service or publicity. Be prepared to show the benefits of the proposed changes. If your suggestions are accepted, work hard to make them work.

Propose a pilot project where a few changes would affect one part of the company. Plan to evaluate the results after three months.

Learn to accept the current working conditions or get another job.

- Negative people at work.

    Negative co-workers can become stressors for you. Chronic complainers, indecisive leaders, overly anxious supervisors, workaholics, or persons who are loud and verbally derogatory toward others all can cause stress.

    If you must work with such persons, learn to tune them out unless it's essential to your own job performance. Get away by yourself during breaks and lunch. Practice stress relieving techniques to help you get through the day. Also develop some rewarding relationships at work that will help balance the negative influences.

- Tedious tasks.

    Every job has tasks that are tedious and boring, but that cannot be avoided. Don't let these become stressors. If you must make copies, collate materials, or address envelopes, set a time goal for yourself and try to meet it. See if you can find a quicker way to get the job done. If you are unable to concentrate in a meeting, make a "to do" list for when you return to your own desk. (However, don't miss important information at the meeting.)

Check Your Job

1. List the *changes* that have occurred in your job over the last 12 months.

2. List the *challenges* (pressures/demands) you face each day that seem to push you beyond your limits.

3. List the *conflicts* that exist and cause stress.

Now look to eliminate some stressors. Resolve or lessen others. Identify those stressors you will have to endure and ask God to increase your coping strength.

Ease Moving Woes

One of the job-related stressors families often face is moving to a new location because of a job transfer or promotion.

Bill Johnson had mixed feelings. His boss informed him of his promotion and transfer to a branch of the company located in a different city. The promotion was welcome. The move was not.

The family also had mixed feelings. Moving is stressful. The cumulative changes add up to a significant number of points on the Social Readjustment Rating Scale (Appendix A). It can be stressful to locate and buy a new house. Tracy will change schools (David will graduate before the move). Bill will face new responsibilities at work. Joanne will need to find a new job and get used to new routines. The family will look for a new church home and adjust to changes in relationships and social activities with friends. There will be changes in routines, shopping locations, doctors, and hundreds of other small adjustments. It can take six months before a family begins to feel comfortable in a new location.

Remember the Israelites? Moses delivered them out of bondage in Egypt and led them to their new home—the Promised Land, flowing with milk and honey. God provided miraculous interventions along the way, giving them daily rations of manna and even bringing them flocks of birds to eat when they cried for meat. Yet their often repeated plea was just to return to Egypt. At least they knew they could survive the old pain. They weren't sure the Promised Land was worth the new pain (Ex. 14:10–12; Num. 11:4–20; 14:1–4; 21:4–5). Yet God remained faithful. He safely led His people home.

Moving can become less stressful if you recognize and prepare for the hassles, minimize the changes whenever possible, plan carefully, and get organized.

- Visit the new location (if possible).

   The Johnsons were blessed because their new location was only 105 miles away. They decided one Saturday to drive to the new city. Bill called a real estate salesperson and arranged for a morning and early afternoon of house hunting. The family made a list of "must haves" and "would likes" for the house in the new town. They packed a picnic lunch, started out early, and enjoyed the day. They selected three houses as possibilities and began working with the realtor on the details.

   Two weeks later the family came back and carefully checked out the neighborhood surrounding the house they hoped to buy. Again they made a list of places to locate: schools, horse stables/trails, beauty shops, grocery stores, gas stations, barber shops, dry cleaners, car repair shops, video rental stores, and fast-food restaurants. These two Saturdays helped the family begin to picture the new location and see themselves functioning in new ways before they actually made the move.

If you can't visit your new location, contact the chamber of commerce for maps and as much other information as you can get, then improvise.

- Plan to keep in touch with the "old" neighborhood.

If your new location is within driving distance of your previous home, make definite plans for return visits. Before you move, set the date to return for dinner, a party, social function, or just a visit. Plan visits for the family and individual members as well.

The Johnsons decided to come back three weeks after their move to spend a day in the old location. After dinner, the family drove home together. It was a long and tiring day, but everyone felt it was worth the effort. And, even though the Johnsons had only been in the new location for three weeks, they discovered that the "old" location wasn't "home" anymore. They were glad to get to their "new" home and sleep in their own beds.

If you keep in touch, and know that you will be returning, you can reduce the stress of moving. If the distance between the two locations is so great that you can't drive back for a day or weekend, then plan for a longer visit after several months.

Regular telephone calls, cards, and letters, as well as visits, can help keep in touch.

• Plan for details.

One of the best things you can do to reduce hassles is to plan for details and get organized.

Label your boxes. No matter how tired you

are when you pack, label all boxes clearly. Mark boxes to tell which room they go into and even into which bureau drawers or kitchen areas. Labeling will help you find specific items when you arrive in the new location.

Don't move excess items. As you pack, sort your possessions into three different stacks: keep, give away, and throw away. Be ruthless. Get rid of anything you don't absolutely need or haven't used in the last five years. You'll never miss it. The less you have to move, the less hassles at both ends of the move.

Pack a tool kit to keep handy for the move. Select several small tools and items you may need when you arrive at the new location. Pack these in a box or tool kit to keep with you in the car for this purpose. You might include tape, scissors, string, pliers, screwdrivers, hammer and nails, picture hangers, light bulbs, matches, flashlight and batteries, toilet paper, pencil, and note paper.

Call ahead to get utilities turned on. Your realtor can provide you with information about turning utilities on, hooking up the telephone, and other necessary services so that when you arrive everything will work and you can immediately begin to settle in.

- Survive the first week.

    The first week in a new location can be stressful. Parents start new jobs, kids start new schools, and virtually everything is new. There are bound to be many ups and downs. Your goal for the first week is not to enjoy yourself, not to feel comfortable and happy, and not to make the cover of "People" magazine as the "All-American Family." Your goal is to survive! The second week you may try for less discomfort and the third week for moments of peace and contentment. Your move is unusual. For most of us it takes a while to settle in.

- Get involved in the new neighborhood.

    Introduce yourself to your neighbors, attend church, and slowly get involved in community activities. You will surprise yourself at how well you can cope in your new surroundings.

- Practice positive self talk.

    Watch what you say to yourself. If you constantly say, "I don't want to be here!" you will have a hard time adjusting. Instead, pick out those parts of the new location that are pleasing to you and tell yourself, "I like the new job, grocery store, school, (or whatever)." Tell yourself "I am beginning to feel comfortable here."

- Put your stress reactivity to work.

    When you begin to experience stress reactivity, do something physical. Unpack boxes, reorganize a closet, cook a special treat, or work in the yard. Put your excess energy to good use.

- Pray.

    Ask God to assist you in adjusting to the new place. He will work things out for you and your family. Here are a few promises from God's Word:

    > For strength: Deuteronomy 33:25; Isaiah 40:29–31
    >
    > For ability: Philippians 4:13; Matthew 19:26
    >
    > For hope: Romans 8:28; 1 Corinthians 1:9
    >
    > For endurance: Isaiah 43:2; Isaiah 41:10
    >
    > For rest: Matthew 11:28; 1 Peter 5:7

- Talk about your feelings.

    At least once a week, talk with your family. Tell each other how you are feeling, what is hard about the adjustment, and what you miss about the old routines and lifestyle. Don't forget to end the discussion with a focus on the good things about the new location, job, school, church, and lifestyle. Talking out the negative feelings will help.

    If you face a move, take time to identify the changes, challenges, and conflicts ahead for you and your family. Follow the formula to identify and study those that can be reduced or eliminated. Take the appropriate actions to make the move less stressful for all of you.

7
✤ Enjoy Family Relationships

Joanne silently cleared the dishes from the table. It had been a difficult evening meal. She and the children were all in such bad moods, Joanne knew they would end up fighting if they stayed in the same room. So she sent David on an errand, told Tracy to do her homework, and politely declined help from Bill. Instead she worked in the kitchen by herself. "Why are family relationships so difficult?" she wondered as she loaded the dishwasher. "We genuinely love each other, but there are times when we seem to attack one another at the slightest excuse."

The current situation started innocently enough at dinner. David talked about his plans for the weekend, and Bill reminded David that he needed to help with the planned chores before he could go off with his buddies. David became angry and resentful. Tracy joined into the ensuing argument, and Joanne's stomach churned so badly she couldn't finish her meal. She added fuel to the family fire by accusing all of them of deliberately spoiling the dinner hour and not appreciating what a great meal she had prepared. Now everyone was upset.

Family relationships can be stressful. Very stressful! We'll just explore a few of the reasons.

Parenting Is an Awesome Responsibility

The Scriptures are filled with admonitions aimed at parents. Parents are expected to teach their children how to take care of themselves and how to live peaceably in a social world. Parents also must teach children the laws and precepts of God. We are charged not to provoke children to anger but to bring them up in the nurture and admonition of the Lord (Deut. 6:7; Prov. 22:6; Eph. 6:4). Our children need our protection, instruction, modeling, encouragement, affirmation, discipline, and guidance. Parenting is demanding. It's no wonder there are times when parents experience frustration and stress.

Joanne worked around the kitchen—she cleaned the counters, put away leftovers, and took meat out of the freezer to thaw for the next day. She still felt hurt and angry. Unbidden, the thought crossed Joanne's mind, "Why did I ever have kids in the first place?" She was shocked at the question.

Don't be shocked, Joanne. You would be surprised at the number of parents who find themselves questioning the joys of parenthood from time to time. Being a parent isn't easy. And often we add to the stress of being parents through our expectations, actions, and reactions. Here are a few steps that can help parents enjoy parenting more than perhaps they have in the past.

- Let children be children.

Once, when David was only 8, Joanne lectured him about forgetting his new jacket at school. David looked up at her and innocently reminded, "But Mom, I can't help it. I'm just a little boy!" And he was right.

Sometimes parents expect adult behavior from children and become very frustrated when all they see is childlike behavior. It's hard enough for an adult to act as an adult. Parents need to allow their children to experience and enjoy their childhoods. This doesn't mean that children are unaccountable or undisciplined. It simply means that our expectations mustn't be unrealistic.

What expectations do you have for your children? If expectations are too high, you place extra stressors in your life because your children may not be able to meet your expectations. Decide to expect the best from your children, but understand that it will be a *child's* best.

God gives us a similar consideration in our spiritual lives. Those who are spiritually immature are encouraged to feast on the "milk" of the Bible in order to grow into spiritual maturity (1 Peter 2:2). As we grow, God enables us to make better decisions and live according to more difficult standards. God accepts where we are in our spiritual journey while at the same time encouraging us to develop in our spiritual growth (Heb. 5:12–14; Eph. 4:14–16).

- Don't live through your children.

Bill felt very disappointed when David didn't go out for baseball in high school. Bill had always wanted to be a baseball player himself and hadn't been able to play. He was wise enough to understand, however, that David couldn't live out his father's fantasies.

Sometimes the dreams do coincide. King David would say he was blessed in this respect with one of his sons. David wanted to build a temple for the Lord, but God said no. David was allowed to gather the materials for the building of the temple and his son, Solomon, was the builder. Solomon fulfilled his father's dreams.

- Let your children know the real you.

Joanne remembers an incident when Tracy, then age 5, came into the living room and saw her mom giggling with a girlfriend. Tracy stood staring for a long time. Joanne wiped the tears from her eyes and asked Tracy, "What's wrong?"

"Nothing," Tracy replied. "I just never saw you laugh like that before."

Joanne realized that she had worked so hard at being a good parent, always teaching, always lecturing, always scolding, always so serious, that her children had never gotten to know her as a genuine person. From that day on she consciously tried to be real with her children.

It's really okay if our children see us cry, laugh, get angry, and experience other genuine emotions. It is one way we can model how to handle ourselves appropriately. Paul reminds us that when we feel angry, we should resolve issues—and not go to bed angry with one another (Eph. 4:26).

- Teach godly values, but understand that the children will choose for themselves as they grow up.

When you teach values, it is important to verbally share them with the children: Explain the whys and wherefores; model the values in your own life; explore together what God has to say about those values; allow open discussion of the values you hold as well as alternative values. Encourage children to consider the consequences of following the alternate values.

Even when parents do their best, some children will choose the worst. To hold yourself responsible and blame yourself for a child's poor choices will add unnecessarily to your stress. Your broken heart will provide stress enough.

Remember King David? His son, Absalom, was a beloved son. But Absalom lived an evil life. Absalom killed his half brother, left the country to escape punishment, and returned to undermine his father's authority as king. Absalom stole the hearts of the people away from David and led them in war against David. But David never gave up. He expected and longed for Absalom to be a good man who would live according to the commandments of the Lord. When Absalom was killed, David wept bitterly—not only for his lost son, but for his lost dreams for his son (2 Sam. 13:23–18:33).

- Share your faith.

One exciting aspect of parenting is sharing your faith in God with your children. Parents have the opportunity to teach children about God's faithfulness, forgiveness, and love. Imagine how happy Lois and Eunice felt when their son and grandson, Timothy, followed God's teachings and was recognized as a child of faith (2 Tim. 1:5).

Remember, you are not accountable for the choices your children make, but you are to let them know about your own relationship with God and how it makes a difference in your life.

- Teach children life skills.

    When David was only 11, Bill and Joanne listed skills he would need in order to function as an adult on his own. They systematically taught David those skills, appropriate to his age level. By the time David was 18 he had mastered all of the basic knowledge, skills, and abilities he needed.

    If you fail to teach your children to cook, clean, do laundry, mend clothes, iron, balance a checkbook, live on a budget, or any of the other basic living skills, they may fail to learn them on their own. Consequently, they will be dependent upon you longer than necessary. Your frustration level will be high if you see your child failing as a young adult.

- Keep house rules consistent.

    Keep house rules to a minimum and your enforcement consistent. Consequences work best if directly related to the infraction so that children see a correlation between the two.

    When you discipline children, remember the purpose of discipline is to train children to do right. Therefore, good discipline not only includes consequences when rules are broken but also compliments when things are done correctly.

Avoid power struggles as much as possible. Too often parents set themselves up for trouble by engaging in power struggles. Remember children will always test set limits. They will always fight to win power games. The books listed at the end of this chapter can help you establish effective communication styles, set house rules and consequences, and eliminate power struggles.

- Be gentle on yourself.

  Do you also have a spouse, a job, and other friendships? These all need and deserve your attention. Take time out from parenting to work on yourself and further develop your own character. Take time to stretch and grow.

  Be the best parent you can, but set realistic expectations for yourself. If expectations are too high, you will fail, and that will add unnecessarily to your stress.

Coordinating Family Times Can Be Challenging

From the time the children were small, Bill and Joanne reserved one evening a week for the family. No outside commitments were allowed to interfere with their family time, and rarely was a change of evening negotiated—except for the times when Bill went out of town for business.

As the children grew older and became more involved with their friends, it became more difficult to retain the integrity of that special evening schedule. On different occasions, David or Tracy needed to be somewhere else on family night. Bill and Joanne did their best to keep "family night" alive, but it was not easy.

As hard as it is to do, parents who resolve to keep one night a week reserved just for family find that the payoff is well worth the trouble. Families can develop intimacy, open communication, and share history. Family night affirms that family commitments are as important as other commitments.

Family nights are intended to be instructive, inspirational, and, most of all, fun. Include games, conversation, projects, sharing, encouragement, research, and other enjoyable activities. Let your children know that they are important to you, not only by your words, but by your actions (1 John 3:18).

When Family Members Are Added

Bill hung up the telephone thoughtfully and looked over at Joanne. He didn't know how to tell her the news. "Honey," he said, "we have to talk." Putting his arm around her shoulders, he led her to the kitchen where they could be alone. Bill told Joanne about his telephone conversation with his aunt.

Bill's mother died a couple years ago, and Bill's father lived alone. According to Bill's aunt, the family must decide how to care for Bill's father. He could be alone for several hours, but needed to be reminded to take his medications, take baths, and eat meals. He could no longer live alone. Bill's father simply refused the retirement center option, and that was beyond Bill's financial resources as well. Although it was going to be a strain, Bill wanted to bring his father into his home.

Bill and Joanne talked about the issues involved in adding a new member to their household. The stressors were many. There would be less privacy, a space problem, conflicts over how things ought to be done, a disruption in the family routine, and changes in the interactions the Johnsons had established among themselves. There would also be additional expense. It was not going to be easy.

It never is easy to accept new members into the family, even when their arrivals are welcomed. New members may include a new spouse, children from previous marriages, children of relatives, relatives who are destitute, older relatives (parents, grandparents, aunts, and uncles), grown children who move back, friends who need help, or strangers who pay for room and board.

When new members arrive, existing family members must make adjustments—and some are not desirable. Sharing limited bathrooms, giving up individual bedrooms, converting family rooms into extra bedrooms, negotiating which television programs to watch, cooking different menus, living with a loss of privacy—these can all cause a high degree of stress reactivity. With careful planning and a positive attitude, you can learn to accept new family members without experiencing stress overload.

When I think of this problem, I am reminded of the widow at Zarephath. God sent Elijah to her during a time of drought in Israel (1 Kings 17:8–16). When Elijah approached the widow, she was gathering sticks to make a fire. She planned to make one last cake from her remaining meal and oil. With no other resources, she knew she and her son would soon starve to death. Elijah told the widow not to worry, but share her meal with him. God would provide for them. Elijah joined the widow's family for the duration of the drought, and God worked a miracle. He made the meal and oil last the whole time. What a hardship it may have seemed when Elijah first asked the widow for a meal, but what an opportunity for God to work a miracle.

- Accept the person as sent from God.

   The first step is to accept the new family member(s) as sent from God—not as an imposition. Pray that God will show you how to minister to the new member and give you a love and patience for that person. Sometimes the new member will only be with the family for a short period of time. Ask God what impact you can have, and how you can best minister to the new family member. Ask God to bless your time together and build a strong, loving relationship.

Remember the slave, Onesimus? He robbed his master, fled to Rome, and was converted by Paul's teachings. In a sense, Onesimus became a member of Paul's family (although Paul was in prison). Paul says he would have liked to keep Onesimus with him in Rome, but instead sent him back to Philemon, his master. God blessed Paul's time with Onesimus. The Spirit worked through Paul to change Onesimus' heart (Philemon 1:10–20).

- Evaluate the living arrangements.

  When you add a new family member, you will want to reevaluate the use of space in your house. Whenever possible, let family members retain their own rooms. This might mean converting the family room, the den, the library, or the garage into an extra living space for the new member. If this is absolutely impossible, you should at the very least give the new member a space that is distinctively his/her own. This might be a closet, a bureau, or a corner of a bedroom.

When the woman from Shunem decided to provide for the prophet Elisha, she asked her husband to build a little chamber off their house where Elisha could have a bed, table, stool, and a candlestick—a place of his own (2 Kings 4:8–11).

- Discuss house rules.

When Bill's dad came to live with the Johnsons, he was shocked to discover that the family didn't eat breakfast together. He tried to change the routine so everyone could be together, but it never worked. Finally Bill and Joanne realized they needed to talk with Dad. They explained how the family agreed on getting together each evening for dinner and each member would have breakfast (or not have breakfast) as his/her schedule dictated.

This discussion resulted in an evening-long meeting. Everyone amicably discussed the house rules and schedules. Bill's dad made suggestions—a few were adopted and worked well for the entire family. Most adjustments were made by Bill's dad.

- Make time to be alone, together.

When Grandpa came to live with the Johnsons, they had to readjust family routines to ensure that there was still time for each person to be alone, and for different people to be together. Bill and Joanne went to their bedroom a half hour earlier so they could be alone together. (Bill's dad stayed in the family room as long as they did at night.) Bill and Joanne also instituted a family "lunch out" once a month, without Bill's dad, so just the four of them could be alone together.

- Use good interpersonal skills.

    It is important that you use the interpersonal skills discussed in chapter 4 when communicating with the new family member. Failure to do so may result in your feeling attacked, pushed, crowded, unappreciated, frustrated, or upset. These stressors will trigger a stress response. You can control your stress response by dealing effectively with the issues as they arise.

A new family member can be a blessing or a curse. What you tell yourself about the experience and how you respond to situations will determine the outcome of the experience. If the arrangement becomes impossible, in spite of everything you do to make it work, it may become necessary to make other arrangements. But first, give it your best shot. Ask God to make the experience a blessing for all concerned.

Sometimes Family Members Leave

Losing a family member can be just as stressful

as gaining a family member. The most common "loss" occurs when children grow up and leave home. Whether they go away to college, move out on their own, or get married, family relationships will experience a significant change.

As older children move out, the role of oldest-child-at-home passes to the next child. Suddenly, this child changes. Some may imitate the sibling who left. Some, having waited for years, "take over" and do things differently. Some children blossom as if their real personalities had been suppressed or over-powered by the dominance of the older brother or sister. Whatever the change, the family may experience stress in adjusting to the various changes in relationships.

Major Trauma Causes Major Stress

Serious injury or illness within the family will add to everyone's stress load. Expect significant changes within the family routine. Added duties of patient care and financial drain (both in medical expense and possible loss of income) affect the whole family.

A robbery, mugging, or rape of a family member can threaten the entire family structure. Members need to depend upon the family strength to stick together and support one another.

The death of a family member causes deep grief

among the remaining members. It is impossible to say which is most difficult—a sudden unexpected death or the loss of a family member after a long-term illness. In all cases, there is family trauma and need for recovery.

Divorce (which is another stressor itself) is sometimes the result of family crises. There are many books available to help people through these difficult situations. (One of these is *Life after Divorce* by Bobbie Reed, CPH, 1993.)

Surviving a major trauma is a challenge. Family members will want to pay close attention to chapter 2 (developing coping strengths) and incorporate these recommendations into their lives. It takes a great deal of strength—physical, mental, spiritual, psychological, and social—to get through major stressors. It's reassuring to know that God is our refuge and strength (Ps. 46:1).

Role Changes Mean Making Adjustments

Parenting presents a series of role changes. When you first bring home a baby son, he depends upon you for everything. You must feed, change, protect, and love the baby. That baby boy needs you desperately and completely.

The bittersweet part of parenting is teaching the child independence—in effect, working yourself out of a job. You teach the boy to roll over, crawl, stand, walk, feed himself, talk for himself, dress himself, take care of himself, make decisions, and so on. As the years go by, your role as parent changes from total protector and provider to teacher, guide, disciplinarian, counselor, friend, and, eventually, associate (when the son becomes a man).

Some of the role changes are difficult. As much as you want your children to grow up and make the right life choices, the process includes a pulling away from you and from dependence upon you. That pulling away, the development of independence, creates conflict. It's a challenge to find the delicate balance between allowing children the freedom to spread their wings and still maintaining proper control as parents.

At the other end of the spectrum comes the role change inherent in caring for aging parents. There comes a reversal in roles that is not usually comfortable at first. When parents are unable to care for themselves, unable to make decisions, and unable to cope with life's frustrations, or when they become too ill to be alone, the adult child must step in and assume the role of protector and sometimes provider, instructor, and guide.

It is never easy to see one's parents decline physically or mentally. It is not easy to decide when to step in and exercise authority, especially when the parent refuses to admit a problem. How long should the older parent exercise freedom of choice? This is a decision each person will have to make for him/herself.

Resolve the Challenges, Relieve the Stress

Take a look at the relationships in your family. Together make a list of *changes, challenges,* and *conflicts* you face. Eliminate those stressors you can. Make plans to reduce the stress reactivity for those stressors you cannot eliminate. When you reduce the strength of stressors in your family life, you are freed to fully enjoy those relationships.

Gordon, Thomas. *Parent Effectiveness Training.* New York: Wyden, 1975.

Gaulke, Earl. *You Can Have a Family Where Everybody Wins.* St. Louis: Concordia Publishing House, 1975.

8
Prepare for Retirement

David cleaned his room. Tracy dusted all the down-stairs rooms in the house. Joanne baked two pies, a cake, three dozen cookies, and a ham. Bill mowed and trimmed the lawn. The Johnsons expected company. Joanne's parents planned to arrive the next morning. As she worked in the kitchen, Joanne thought about her parents, and once again mentally applauded them for being wise enough to prepare for retired life.

It's never too early to prepare for your retirement years. The statistics for those who don't prepare are grim. The sudden change from working to nonworking; from a lifelong routine to a nonroutine; and from constant demands to freedom can be a major change—an unbearable stress. Some people become bored, physically ill, and some actually die within a very short time after retirement. Don't let this happen to you.

Plan to Be Solvent

Start a retirement savings account as soon as

you start working. If you don't have a retirement savings account, start one today. As soon as you have enough money saved to invest in a safe place, do so. Never stop saving, even if you put away only a little each month.

In addition to establishing a savings account, eliminate your debts. Resolve to pay off your car and home loans. For details about planning a financially secure future, consult the various books available.

Live modestly. Don't live up to your total income; definitely don't exceed your total income. Learn to live on about 70% of your net income (income after taxes). Give 10% to God. Invest 10% and save 10%. If you are faithful and stick to this plan, you will be well ahead financially when your retirement date comes.

Plan to Be Active

Plan to be active—physically, mentally, and spiritually—after retirement. It's easy to become a "couch potato"—get up late, sip coffee or tea all day, take an afternoon nap, watch television, have dinner, and go to bed early.

Make an exhaustive list of things you would like to do but for which you have not made time. Make a list of activities you enjoy but that you have not had time to do as frequently as you would like. Finally, make a list of things you do now and plan to keep on doing when you retire.

Start a list of books to read, music to listen to, videos to view, places you want to visit, people you want to get to know better, clubs or groups you want to join.

In order to be active in your retirement, start now. Keep yourself in good physical condition. Develop and maintain your physical coping strength in the ways outlined in chapter 2.

Plan to Be Productive

It's possible to be active without being productive. Part of your retirement plan will include finding ways in which you can be productive. Perhaps you like to work on crafts, quilt, can fruits and vegetables, or some other productive activity. These may have been too time consuming to do while working full time. Retirement will be a great time to develop or rediscover these skills and put them to work.

Perhaps there is a way you can use the knowledge and skills you developed in your job to help others. The organization called SCORE may have a chapter in your town. This organization uses retired business persons to serve as consultants to small businesses. It always feels good to be able to "give back."

You may want to start a small business of your own when you retire. You could buy and sell, provide a service, or coordinate the services of others.

Retirement may be the time to teach at the community college level or in an adult education program. What about volunteering as a literacy instructor and help adults learn to read? Hospitals can always use volunteers. Maybe your church needs extra hands to fold and stuff Sunday bulletins, address envelopes, or type letters.

Each Christian is given spiritual gifts. Perhaps you have not yet made full use of your gifts. Retirement may be just the time to become more active in the work of the ministry, making full use of the gifts and talents God has given you.

Plan to Be Fulfilled

You may be active and productive and still not feel fulfilled. Therefore, you need to identify those things which affirm you and fulfill your needs. Productivity gives some people a sense of fulfillment. Acting or painting helps others feel fulfilled. Studying and learning are still other ways to find inner excitement.

Would you like to enroll in a class at a local seminary or Bible school? Do you dream of writing a book? Do you want to go on short-term mission trips? What dreams have not been realized? Is there a way you can do those things when you retire? Probably.

Plan to Be Content

Life does not always turn out as we plan. We can get closer to our goals if we plan in the direction we want to go.

If, after all is said and done, things fall short of our expectations, we can, with the Spirit's encouragement, be content. If we cannot change our situation, we must, with God's help, accept reality. The apostle Paul provided us a terrific example through his life. Paul's life was a series of extremes. He had been revered and reviled. He was hungry and had plenty. He was comfortable and experienced a ship wreck. Paul experienced poverty and abundance. Paul told Timothy that godliness with contentment was great gain, and that as long as we have food and clothing, we can be content (1 Tim. 6:6–8). In Hebrews God reminds us not to covet what others have but to be content with whatever we have (13:5).

Contentment is different from resignation. If you feel resigned, you may feel bitter. If you are content, you trust God to provide the necessities for your life. Ask the Holy Spirit to give you a contented and grateful heart.

Don't Fail to Plan

No matter how you desire to spend your retirement days, don't forget to plan ahead of time. This is one way to avoid the stress the changes will bring. Use our formula:

1. Make a list of anticipated *changes* retirement will bring to your life.

2. Make a list of the *challenges* (pressures, demands) retirement will bring to your life.

3. Make a list of *conflicts* you anticipate during your retirement.

Plan ways to eliminate as many of the stressors as possible. Take steps to reduce your stress reactivity in the areas you have identified. Develop ways to compensate for the stress you anticipate in your retirement lifestyle. Never stop working to develop your coping strengths. Your retirement years can truly be golden.

✤ CONCLUSION

You Don't Have to be Stressed Out

As we stated when we began, life is stressful. You cannot avoid change, challenges, or conflicts. Use the principles in this book. You can learn to identify the basic and major stressors in your life. You can begin to eliminate some of the stressors you face. You can control your stress reactivity to some extent, and most importantly, you can develop your coping strength. In actuality, your experiences will make you strong! You will have truly transformed your stress into strength.

God stands ready to lift you up in times of joy and times of stress. Through the redeeming work of His Son, He forgives the wrong decisions you make in times of stress and sets you on the right path. Life is stressful, but don't be stressed out!

APPENDIX A

Social Readjustment Rating Scale

Dr. Thomas Holmes and colleagues at the University of Washington School of Medicine developed this Social Readjustment Rating Scale that is widely used to determine susceptibility to disease.

As you can see, the scale lists 43 life events and gives each a weighted point value. An accumulated point value of 150–199 in one year indicates a mild problem, a 37% chance of experiencing physical symptoms of illness. Scores from 200–299 suggest a moderate problem with a 51% chance of stress overload and physical illness. A score of more than 300 indicates a high probability of serious illness unless a person has significantly developed coping strengths to deal with increased stress.

Add up the score of the life events listed below that have occurred in your life during the last 12 months. If an event has happened more than once, you add points for that item as many times as it occurred. If there has been a significant stressor in your life in the last 12 months that does not appear on the chart, decide how it would compare with the life events that are listed. Assign the event an appropriate point value.

RANK • LIFE EVENT	MEAN VALUE
1. Death of a Spouse	100
2. Divorce	73
3. Marital Separation	65
4. Jail Term	63
5. Death of Close Family Member	63
6. Personal Injury or Illness	53
7. Marriage	50
8. Fired at Work	47
9. Marital Reconciliation	45
10. Retirement	45
11. Change in Health of Family Member	44
12. Pregnancy	40
13. Sex Difficulties	39
14. Gain of New Family Member	39
15. Business Readjustment	39
16. Change in Financial State	38
17. Death of Close Friend	37
18. Change to Different Line of Work	36
19. Change in Number of Arguments with Spouse	35
20. Mortgage over $10,000	31
21. Foreclosure of Mortgage or Loan	30

Reprinted with permission from *Journal of Psychosomatic Research*, Vol. 11, Homes/Rahe, "The Social Readjustment Rating Scale," (1967), Elsevier Science Ltd., Pergamon Imprint, Oxford, England.

APPENDIX B

Selected Bibliography

Bright, Bill and Vonette. *Managing Stress in Marriage: Help for Couples on the Fast Track*. Nashville: Thomas Nelson Publishers, Inc., 1990.

Burton, Arnold. *Helping Kids Cope: A Parents' Guide to Stress Management*. Elgin: David C. Cook Publishing Company, 1992.

Evans, W. Glyn. *Don't Quit Until You Taste the Honey*. Nashville: Broadman Press, 1993.

Greenberg, Jerrold S. *Comprehensive Stress Management*. Dubuque: Brown and Benchmark, 1993.

Hart, Archibald D. *Adrenalin and Stress*. Dallas: Word, Inc., 1991.

Lewis, Deborah S. *Motherhood Stress*. Grand Rapids: Zondervan Publishing House, 1992.

Lush, Jean and Pam Vredevelt. *Women & Stress*. Ada: Baker Book House, 1992.

Malony, H. Newton. *Relaxation for Christians*. New York: Ballantine Books, Inc., 1992.

Manning, George. *Stress without Distress*. Dallas: South-Western Publishing Co., 1988.

Menconi, Peter et al. *Stressed Out: Keeping It Together When It's Falling Apart*. Colorado Springs: NavPress, 1988.

Morell, Paul L. *Living in the Lions' Den: How to Cope with Life's Stress*. Nashville: Abingdon Press, 1992.

Sehnert, Keith W. *Stress-Unstress*. Minneapolis: Augsburg Fortress, 1981.

Sprinkle, Patricia H. *Women Who Do Too Much: Stress & The Myth of the Superwoman*. Grand Rapids: Zondervan Publishing House, 1992.